Practical Physiotherapy for Small Animal Practice

Practical Physiotherapy for Small Animal Practice

David Prydie
Isobel Hewitt

WILEY Blackwell

Library of Congress Cataloging-in-Publication Data

Prydie, David, author.
    Practical physiotherapy for small animal practice / David Prydie, Isobel Hewitt.
        p. ; cm.
    Includes bibliographical references and index.
        ISBN 978-1-118-66154-3 (paper)
    I. Hewitt, Isobel, author. II. Title.
    [DNLM: 1. Physical Therapy Modalities–veterinary. 2. Hospitals, Animal–standards. 3. Musculoskeletal Diseases–veterinary. 4. Physical Therapy Specialty–methods. SF 925]
    SF925.P78 2015
    636.089'582–dc23

                                                                        2015018215

A catalogue record for this book is available from the British Library.

Wiley also publishes its books in a variety of electronic formats. Some content that appears in print may not be available in electronic books.

Set in 9/12pt Meridien by SPi Global, Chennai, India

Printed in the UK

Contents

Contents

v

About the authors

DAVID PRYDIE
BVMS, CertSAO, CCRT, MRCVS

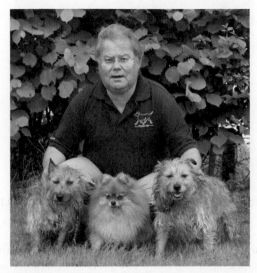

David Prydie with his two terrier crosses Spud and Sprout, and his Pomeranian, Mr. Darcy.

David graduated from Glasgow veterinary school in 1981 and obtained his certificate in Small Animal Orthopaedics in 1991. He has worked in first opinion and orthopaedic referral practice throughout the United Kingdom. In 2009, David obtained his Certificate in Canine Rehabilitation from The Canine Rehabilitation Institute, USA. He currently owns and runs Physio-Vet, a dedicated small animal physiotherapy practice in Cheshire, Crewe, UK (www.physio-vet.co.uk). David has lectured on animal rehabilitation and physiotherapy at many national and international conferences. His particular interests are canine sports medicine and the management of chronic musculoskeletal diseases, such as canine osteoarthritis and degenerative myelopathies.

Isobel Hewitt
BSc (Hons,) MSc, ACPAT (Cat A)

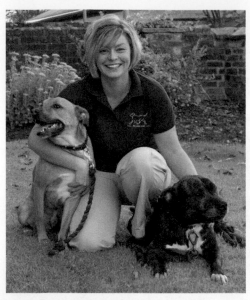

Isobel Hewitt with her Staffordshire Bull Terrier Wilson and her Staffy Cross Marley.

Isobel graduated in physiotherapy in 2003 from Sheffield Hallam University. She is a Chartered Physiotherapist and has many years of experience as a human physiotherapist. She has her own human physiotherapy practice specialising in musculoskeletal physiotherapy. In 2009, she completed her MSc in Animal Physiotherapy from the Royal Veterinary College, London. She has worked at Physio-Vet since its opening. Her special interests are proprioceptive retraining, orthotic and splinting devices and functional rehabilitation for small animals.

She is a category A member of ACPAT (Association of Chartered Physiotherapists in Animal Therapy).

Preface

Physiotherapy on dogs and cats has been practiced for well over 25 years. The benefits for patients and practices have been clearly demonstrated. This said, there is still little undergraduate training and the majority of practices offer little or no physiotherapy. A lot of people within the profession are aware of physiotherapy but are not quite sure what it involves.

This textbook is aimed at veterinary surgeons, veterinary nurses and others who want to know more about physiotherapy in small animals. These people may be considering introducing physiotherapy to their practice or considering a training course. We have tried to explain what physiotherapy is and how it is of benefit to the animal, owner and practice. For those who want more details and evidence of the benefits of physiotherapy in small animals, please refer to the Further Readings section (Appendix 3).

We have written this textbook from a practical point of view with advice on selection of equipment, examination, treatment protocols and charging. Our writings and recommendations are based on the cases that we see and treat on a daily basis. We have included chapters on healing and anatomy as they form the basis of treatment protocols and examination. The textbook is by no means definitive and it is important for each therapist to develop his/her own examination and treatment protocols. However, this can only be done with experience of cases. This textbook offers a starting place that can then be adapted and built upon.

David Prydie
Isobel Hewitt

Acknowledgements

The authors would like to thank all the staff, clients and patients of the Physio-Vet Clinic in Crewe, UK. We would especially like to thank Lydia Critchlow for her help in taking many of the photos. Special thanks also go to Keith Hague for his fantastic drawings. We would like to thank all the people who have sent us pictures for use in this textbook.

David would like to thank Stuart Carmichael for his pictures, help and advice while writing this textbook. David would especially like to thank his wife, Lorna, for her patience and support over the last year.

Isobel would like to thank her family, friends and colleagues, especially Andraya Hiscock and Mark Humphreys for their support, help and motivational talks when required.

David Prydie would like to dedicate this textbook to the memory of his parents. His father, Jack, was also a veterinary surgeon and one of the pioneers in the development of small animal vaccines, died in 1988. David's mother, Nan, died in the last week of writing this textbook.

Acknowledgements

The authors would like to thank all the staff, clients and patients of the Physio-Vet Clinic in Crowe, UK. We would especially like to thank Lydia Cuthb?? for her help in taking many of the photos. Special thanks also go to Keith Blake for his fantastic drawings. We would like to thank all the people who have sent us pictures for use in this textbook.

David would like to thank Stuart Carmichael for his pictures, help and advice while writing this textbook. David would especially like to thank his wife, Lorna, for her patience and support over the last year.

Isobel would like to thank her family, friends and colleagues, especially Andrea Bacon and Mark Humphreys for their support, help and motivational talks when required.

David Prydie would like to dedicate this textbook to the memory of his parents. His father, Jack, was also a veterinary surgeon and one of the pioneers to the development of small animal vaccine, died in 1988. David's mother, Mary, died in the last week of writing this textbook.

About the companion website

Practical Physiotherapy for Small Animal Practice is accompanied by a companion website:

www.wiley.com/go/practical-physiotherapy-for-small-animals

The website includes:
- Client education handouts.

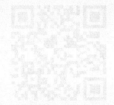

CHAPTER 1

Introduction

All professions develop and evolve as new research is conducted; pioneering techniques become everyday techniques and in veterinary medicine, the use of physiotherapy to complement current treatments is becoming more widely recognised and utilised. Many owners are becoming more aware of physiotherapy through magazines, dog training clubs, social media and word of mouth that often they seek out physiotherapists and are asking whether it could be beneficial for their pets. Physiotherapy must always be carried out after a veterinary consultation and with veterinary consent. It is important to seek out appropriately qualified practitioners to carry out physiotherapy in order to ensure that no harm will come to animals during treatment. This textbook aims to introduce physiotherapy, discussing and outlining its basic principles.

Physiotherapy is defined as the therapeutic use of physical agents or means, such as massage or exercises, to treat disease or injury. It is an extremely useful adjunct to medicine, human and veterinary. The aim is to restore mobility/function and quality of life to patients. This is done by stimulating the healing process to restore injured tissues, improve the balance/strength of the injured tissues and stabilising the cardiorespiratory, neurological and musculoskeletal systems. Physiotherapy also has an important role in optimising performance and injury prevention in sporting and working animals. It can be performed on any animal, but the majority of cases seen in small animal practice are dogs.

Physiotherapy is often used to correct complications that may have occurred as a result of surgery; however, if introduced early and appropriately, these complications can be avoided. The rehabilitation must be of the highest standard to fulfill the expectations of owners and veterinarians alike. For example, following TTA surgery, physiotherapy will aid correct gait re-education-whereas without physiotherapy, the animal may adopt an adaptive gait pattern.

Physiotherapy can be beneficial for animals in a wide range of conditions. Traditionally, physiotherapy is divided into a wide variety of specialties. In veterinary medicine, we could see the following divisions:

- Musculoskeletal.
- Respiratory.
- Orthopaedics.
- Neurological.
- Sports medicine.

Practical Physiotherapy for Small Animal Practice, First Edition.
Edited by David Prydie and Isobel Hewitt.
© 2015 John Wiley & Sons, Ltd. Published 2015 by John Wiley & Sons, Ltd.
Companion Website: www.wiley.com/go/practical-physiotherapy-for-small-animals

- Elderly care/geriatrics.
- Developmental problems.

Musculoskeletal: Most people consider this as 'traditional physiotherapy'. The conditions seen can be split into soft-tissue injuries, such as sprains/strains or ruptures of ligament, tendon or muscle; bursitis and bone or joint injuries, such as fractures (Figure 1.1) or joint disease, such as OCD. The injuries may be a result of either a traumatic event or overuse, where the owner cannot recall the specific onset of symptoms.

Respiratory: This is the acute care of animals in hospital; it could be post-anaesthetic recovery or ventilated animals. Physiotherapy is aimed to manage secretions, prevent pressure sores, prevent atelectasis, reduce the work of breathing and optimise the ventilation/perfusion ratio to ensure high oxygen saturation levels. These aims are achieved using positioning (for pressure relief, postural drainage or to influence ventilation/perfusion ratio within the lungs), manual techniques such as percussion (Figure 1.2) or vibrations to remove secretions, neuromuscular techniques such as rib springing to increase lung capacity and manual hyperinflation or bagging to improve ventilation and aid secretion removal.

Orthopaedics: Physiotherapy following surgery is used to maximise the success of surgery. By working with the surgeon, the recovery can be optimised. Orthopaedic surgeons may have their own protocols for rehabilitation following surgery and knowledge of these protocols is needed by the owner and therapist before embarking on a rehabilitation programme. These protocols guide the therapist on how much weight can be put through the leg and when different exercises can be introduced.

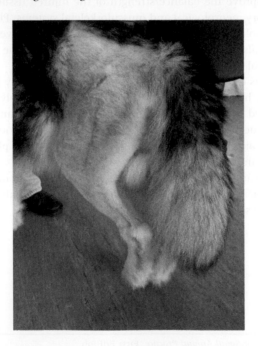

Figure 1.1 *Post fracture.* This picture shows an Alaskan Malamute following a femoral fracture after being kicked by a horse. The main aims of physiotherapy for this dog are to improve its weight bearing on the leg and increase its muscle mass/strength.

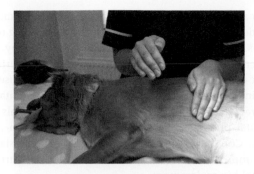

Figure 1.2 *Respiratory physiotherapy*. Following anaesthesia any animals requiring ventilation have the potential to develop retained secretions. Ventilated animals will also be sedated and therefore not move around, which can cause secretions to pool in the lungs and need removal.

Neurological: Neurological physiotherapy is the rehabilitation of the animal following neurological injury, which can involve single limb or whole body. Neurological damage can be managed conservatively or surgically and may completely resolve or can leave lasting damage. The amount of initial damage usually has a significant impact on the amount of recovery that can be achieved. Long-term solutions to permanent damage sometimes have to be sought, such as wheels, harnesses or splints, to support the animal's everyday activities (Figure 1.3).

Sports medicine: The preparation of an animal for athletic activity is extremely important requiring physical training, skill training and cardiovascular training. Physiotherapy can help guide owners on appropriate conditioning programmes for certain sports and specific to the animal being trained. Different sports will place very different demands on a dog, for example, the endurance capability of a sled dog opposed to the speed of a racing greyhound.

The rehabilitation of sports injuries is also extremely important as often these animals are not lame but subtle changes in muscle tightness can affect their performance.

Elderly care/geriatrics: As pets (and owners) are living longer now, there is a high population of arthritic animals seen in clinics; they can often have other

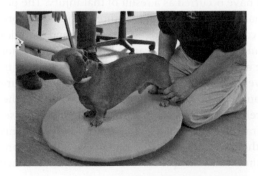

Figure 1.3 *Neurological physiotherapy*. After a neurological event, physiotherapy can aid recovery by providing sensory input and re-education of normal movement.

co-morbidities such as diabetes that can complicate the rehabilitation process. The provision of a holistic approach to managing these animals, using tools such as Aim OA (http://aimoasys.com/why-aim-oa/) will mean they can stay comfortable and functional for longer. The AIM OA website is available for veterinary practices to help provide holistic care for the elderly and arthritic animals. It uses a management strategy encompassing pain relief, exercises, diet and environmental factors.

Developmental problems: A large number of young animals are seen with genetic/developmental problems, and they benefit greatly from physiotherapy to support their joints. Conditions such as hip and elbow dysplasia are often seen. Physiotherapy can improve their quality of life and prevent further problems or surgeries such as total hip replacements.

The benefits of physiotherapy

Physiotherapy can be of benefit to all animals; however, the choice of treatment can be limited by any concurrent disease or illness. The behaviour of an animal, the level of understanding of the owner and their emotions can all influence the success of physiotherapy. For example, a nervous owner will unsettle the animal causing it to become tense which can adversely affect the examination and subsequent treatment session. The objective of physiotherapy is for the animal and the owner to be part of the treatment and it therefore must be as least stressful experience for both of them as possible.

The objectives of a rehabilitation programme are to reduce pain, restore movement, improve gait, increase muscle strength and improve function. From these broad objectives, the formation of a rehabilitation programme will be tailored to suit an individual's situation and take into account the many factors that influence rehabilitation.

The knowledge of the healing process (which is outlined in Chapter 3) can help maximise strength of healing tissues following injury and prevent complications arising from the healing process. This is achieved by giving appropriate physiotherapeutic intervention at an appropriate time.

The examination (which is outlined in Chapter 4) of an animal will help identify not only the injury that it has been referred to physiotherapy for, but also any compensations that have occurred as a result of that injury. The physiotherapist will also assess the animal's conformation and posture as this is the cornerstone for good movement. A poor conformation can tighten muscles, and chronically tight muscles can alter bone alignment, which in turn can complicate rehabilitation. Understanding movement, posture and conformation means the animal will be treated holistically and this can improve the long-term prognosis for an animal (Figures 1.4 and 1.5).

When treating animals, it is also very important to educate the owners on how they can help the rehabilitation process, through a home exercise programme and self-management strategies. It is important to understand the clients' expectations of physiotherapy and their goals/aims for the animal. The introduction of physiotherapy at the appropriate time will often promote the safe return to function or activity at the earliest time.

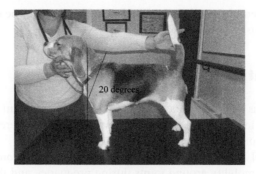

Figure 1.4 *Poor conformation*. This shows poor conformation where the angle of the joints is not ideal leading to muscle imbalance that can cause dysfunction and pain.

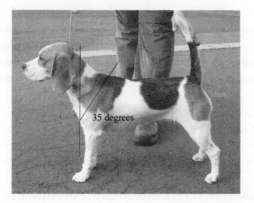

Figure 1.5 *Good conformation*. An animal with good conformation is less likely to have injuries and develop problems as its muscular and skeletal systems are in balance.

In elderly patients or those with a chronic problem, an ongoing physiotherapy programme will maintain the function of an animal for as long as possible. It is particularly useful in these cases to educate the owner on adaptations that can be made in the home environment to support their animal, such as the provision of rugs on slippery floors and placing the animal's bed out of drafts to ensure they do not get cold and stiffen up overnight (in arthritic animals).

Physiotherapists are trained to conduct specific and progressive rehabilitation programmes based on evidence-based treatments. By setting goals throughout the treatment process, the owner (and therapist) can monitor the progress of the animal towards the completion of treatment.

Physiotherapy is used to maintain soundness in competition animals by training owners to be able to recognise signs of reduced performance and educating them on warm ups or stretches for their animals. The provision of competition-specific conditioning programmes for athletic dogs and preseason checks will help to prevent injury. These checks will help to identify any areas of the dog that show subtle changes in range of movement that could be caused by trigger points in the muscle, which, if treated, will not cause loss of performance.

Contraindications

There are numerous contraindications to specific physiotherapeutic techniques and they are addressed individually within the relevant chapters. There are certain conditions where caution should be taken, these include:

Pregnancy – Manual therapies and certain electrotherapies are contraindicated due to the increased mobility around joints during pregnancy and the affect of electrotherapy on growing tissues. It is also worth noting that pregnancy of the owner needs to be known if using pulsed electromagnetic energy.

Cancer – If the patient has known metastatic disease, electrotherapy is contraindicated in that area and is questionable whether it should be used at all. The patient is also likely to fatigue easily, and hence exercise therapy needs to be kept gentle.

Circulation problems – Many physiotherapeutic interventions are used to increase circulation to aid healing. If the circulatory system could not withstand an increase in the area to be treated, then caution should be taken when choosing the treatment method.

Myopathies – Such as myasthenia gravis and exertional rhabdomyolysis need to be recognised and diagnosed by a veterinary surgeon. Physiotherapy is not indicated or appropriate in these cases. If a patient is referred to physiotherapy and is suspected to have a myopathy, prompt referral back to the veterinary surgeon is required.

Behaviour – Aggressive animals need to be treated with extreme caution. The aggression can be a sign of pain, which will reduce as the treatment progresses, however the therapist must be careful to protect him/herself at all times by the use of a muzzle and the owner handling the patient where possible. Some animals can become aggressive when placed in a clinical situation and it is important to recognise this and work with the owner to minimise the stress levels of the animal and work on desensitising the animal to the situation.

It is important to state that when working in rehabilitation, a close relationship between the referring veterinary surgeon, physiotherapist and owner is required. If a case is not responding to physiotherapy, further investigations may be required. For example, a case referred to physiotherapy for stifle pain that is not responding to treatment could be referred lumbar pain from spondylosis of that region.

CHAPTER 2

Anatomy: structure and function of the musculoskeletal system

This chapter aims to give an overview of the structure and function of the musculoskeletal system. Bony landmarks, palpable on the live dog, will be highlighted as they are important for clinical examination and form the reference points for measuring range of motion. In most instances, the location of muscle *groups* will be described. Where specific pathological conditions occur in an *individual muscle, tendon or ligament*, these structures will be described in more detail. For an in-depth guide to anatomy, the readers are referred to more detailed texts (see further reading, Appendix 3).

The structure of a tissue is a result of the forces (function) placed upon it. This is sometimes called adaptive remodelling (Wolff's law.) Originally, this was applied only to bone and can be demonstrated by placing a foreleg in a cast so that the cast takes the weight previously taken by the bone. The bone demineralises and loses some of its strength. This change is reversible by removing the cast and allowing weight-bearing forces to act upon the bone. Wolff's law is equally true for other structures within the musculoskeletal system. The musculoskeletal system is a dynamic system that is designed to move, and its structure depends on that movement. Movement may also influence nutrition, for example, cartilage. Immobilisation can have devastating effects on the musculoskeletal system, but may be necessary to protect sites of injury and surgical repair. Physiotherapy can help reduce the impact of periods of immobilisation or cage rest by maintaining calculated forces and stresses on the musculoskeletal system without compromising the surgical repair or site of injury.

Collagen

Collagen is the main building block in the body and is found in a host of different tissues. There are many types of collagen, but for the purpose of this textbook, we focus on the three main types, which are described as follows:

Type 1 collagen is found in connective tissue and is very strong. It consists of long triple-helix proteins interwoven with adjoining strands that intertwine to form strong rope-like structures with high tensile strength. It is found in tendons, ligaments and bone.

Type 2 collagen consists of shorter chains of proteins than type 1 collagen. The strands are arranged more randomly and in different directions. They are found within the

Practical Physiotherapy for Small Animal Practice, First Edition.
Edited by David Prydie and Isobel Hewitt.
© 2015 John Wiley & Sons, Ltd. Published 2015 by John Wiley & Sons, Ltd.
Companion Website: www.wiley.com/go/practical-physiotherapy-for-small-animals

extracellular matrix of articular cartilage. Type 2 collagen is also a main component of fibrocartilage that is found in the menisci.

Type 3 collagen is found in blood vessels, skin and intestines. It also has a triple-helix structure but with much shorter chains. Type 3 collagen is produced by fibroblasts in response to injury and forms part of the initial scar. Gradually as scar tissue is reorganised, the type 3 collagen is converted to type 1 collagen.

Elastin

Elastin is another protein found in many connective tissues, including tendons, ligaments, joint capsule and cartilage. Elastin allows these tissues to undergo reversible deformity. The amount of elastin in a tissue varies greatly depending upon the degree of elasticity of that tissue. For instance, joint capsules that undergo repeated cycles of elongation and recoil contain significantly more elastin than bone where its presence is restricted mainly to the blood vessels. Elastin is produced during the repair and remodelling phases of tissue healing.

Bone

Bone consists of a type 1 collagen framework with an extracellular matrix of calcium salts (calcium hydroxylapatite and others). In *cortical bone*, as in the shaft of a long bone, the framework is a series of overlapping Haversian units. These have a central blood vessel with concentrically arranged cylinders of bone matrix. Embedded in the bone matrix are the osteocytes that are responsible for the production of the matrix.

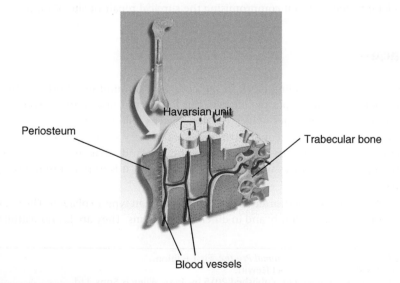

Figure 2.1   Schematic representation of the structure of a long bone showing the Haversian systems, cancellous bone, periosteum, endosteum and bone marrow.

Trabecular or cancellous bone is found at the ends of long bones (metaphysis) and on the endosteal surface of long bones, immediately below the endosteum. Trabecular bone is composed of sheets of bone (trabeculae) surrounding islands of fat and haemopoietic cells. Trabecular bone has a rich blood supply and is populated by large numbers of osteoblasts. The bone is covered by a periosteal surface externally and an endosteal surface in the medullary cavity. The periosteum and endosteum are also rich in blood vessels and osteoblasts. Osteoblasts are responsible for the production of new bone. They lay down the extracellular matrix (ECM) and eventually become embedded in the ECM and mature into osteocytes (Figure 2.1).

Bone is constantly undergoing remodelling and is a balance between the activity of osteoblasts, which lay down new bone and the resorption of the existing bone by osteoclasts. This remodelling activity is controlled by the osteophytes that respond to alteration in the mechanical forces applied to the Haversian systems. The osteocytes then trigger increased osteoblast or osteoclast activity depending on the mechanical forces.

Cartilage

There are three basic types of cartilage.

1 *Hyaline or articular cartilage.* This covers the opposing surfaces of bones making up a synovial joint. Hyaline cartilage consists of an extracellular matrix of proteoglycan with type 2 collagen strands arranged in different directions. It also has some elastin strands. It is sparsely populated by chondrocytes that are responsible for the production of the extracellular matrix. Cartilage is avascular and aneural. Articular cartilage undergoes considerable reversible deforming forces during joint movement. When cartilage is compressed, the cellular matrix loses water and waste products. As it is decompressed, the water and dissolved nutrients return. This is an important mechanism for the nutrition of the chondrocytes. Replenishment of extracellular matrix does occur, but if sufficient articular cartilage damage occurs, repair is with fibrocartilage.

2 *Fibrocartilage.* Fibrocartilage consists of an extracellular matrix with type 1 collagen and elastin. The chondrocytes are embedded in the matrix. Fibrocartilage is a tough flexible tissue, and is found in the menisci, annulus fibrosis of the discs and in entheses (see page 10).

3 Elastic cartilage is very flexible due to its high elastin content. Examples would include the epiglottis, larynx and ears.

Tendons, ligaments and entheses

Both tendons and ligaments are made of dense connective tissue mostly composed of type 1 collagen. They have few cells (fibroblasts) and poor blood supply, and hence the healing process is slow in these tissues (Figure 2.2).

In *tendons*, the fibres are arranged in parallel bundles. Tendons also run in sheaths that facilitate free movement through surrounding tissues.

In *ligaments*, the fibres are less parallel and less closely woven to allow twisting. Ligaments also contain more elastin, therefore allowing for more stretch.

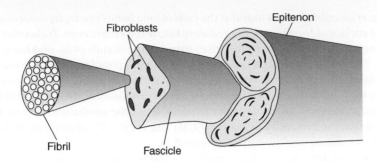

Figure 2.2   Diagrammatic representation of the structure of tendons. BSAVA Manual of Canine and Feline Musculoskeletal Disorders. Figure 8.2, page 110. Reproduced with permission of Samantha Elmhurst.

Entheses

Entheses are specialised structures at the attachment sites of muscles, tendons and ligaments. Entheses have evolved to dissipate the tremendous stresses that occur at the bone/muscle or bone/tendon junction. There are two types of entheses. *Fibrous entheses* occur where muscle attaches directly to bone. Collagen fibres (Sharpey's fibres) run from the muscle, blend into the periosteum and attach to the cortical bone. Fibrocartilage entheses contain a zone of fibrocartilage at the site of the tendon or ligament attachment. These serve as a transition area between the parallel fibres of the tendon or ligament and the bone matrix.

Function of tendons and ligaments

Tendons

Tendon connects muscle to bone and acts to transfer the power generated by the muscle to the leaver action of the bone. Tendons have twice the tensile strength of muscle, and hence often the muscle tears at the musculo-tendon junction.

Ligaments

Ligaments stabilise joints. They connect bone to bone. They guide joint movement. They prevent excess movement of the joint.

Injury of tendons and ligaments

Injury can be a sudden snap due to excessive forces, such as an acute traumatic cranial cruciate rupture. However, more commonly, injuries to tendons and ligaments are repetitive strain injuries. Repetitive overloading of tendons and ligaments causes microfractures and disruption within the collagen bundles.

Factors affecting tendon and ligament injury

Ageing. As animals age, the amount of collagen present in their body decreases.

Immobilisation. If the tendons and ligaments are not used and stressed within normal limits, they become loose and unable to carry out their full function.

Repetitive strain such as contact dismounts in agility dogs can lead to tendon and ligament injury.

Physical training leads to an increase in strength of tendons, thereby reducing the risk of injury.

Joints

Joints are divided into three types as follows:
1 Fibrous joints (synarthroses). These have little or no motion. An example would be the sutures in the bones of the skull and tooth sockets.
2 Cartilaginous joints. These have limited movement that permits compression and stretching. Examples would be
   (a) Hyaline cartilage (synchondrosis) such as costochondral junctions and epiphyseal growth plates in the long bones of growing animals.
   (b) Fibrocartilage (amphiarthrosis) such as mandibular symphysis.
3 Synovial joints (diarthroses). These allow for the greatest range of motion. They consist of two or more bone endings covered with hyaline (articular) cartilage.

Synovial joints have a joint cavity, joint capsule, synovial membrane and synovial fluid. In addition, some joints may have intra-articular ligaments, tendons, menisci and fat pads. Other ligaments and tendons may be extra-articular.

The synovial membrane is very vascular, and blends with the periosteum. It is thrown into numerous villus projections. The function of the synovial membrane is phagocytosis and synovial fluid production.

Synovial fluid is a filtrate of blood to which mucoproteins, such as hyaluronic acid, have been added by the cells of the synovial membrane. The function of the synovial fluid is to lubricate the joint to help reduce wear and tear and to provide nutrition for the chondrocytes in the articular cartilage.

Intervertebral discs

The intervertebral discs lie between the bodies of neighbouring vertebrae with the exception of the atlas and axis. The disc is composed of a tough outer fibrous layer, the annulus fibrosis, which is comprised of fibrocartilage and a jelly-like centre, the nucleus pulposus.

Muscle

Types of muscle
There are three types of muscle found within the body as follows:
- Smooth muscle found in the gut and blood vessels.
- Heart muscle.
- Striated muscles. These are the muscle of conscious movement. The scope of this textbook is restricted to striated muscle.

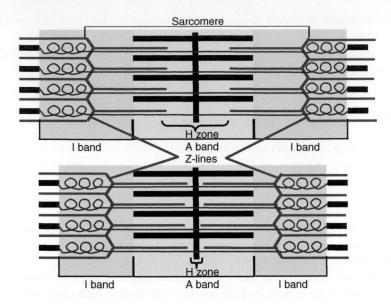

Figure 2.3   Schematic representation of muscle and the sliding filament theory.   Akers and Denbow Anatomy and Physiology of Domestic animals. Figure 7.11. Reproduced with permission of Wiley.

How muscle works

The most popular theory as to how muscle works is the *Sliding Filament Theory* (Figure 2.3).

The myosin molecules have heads. When ATP releases energy, the heads snap up to attach on to the actin. The actin is moved inwards moving the Z-lines towards each other and it results in a shortening of the sarcomere, myofibril and muscle. When the energy has been used, the heads snap back down causing the Z-lines and the actin molecules to return to their original position. Alternating layer of actin and myosin are held together by cross-bridges.

Motor unit

A motor unit consists of a single nerve fibre (neuron) and all the muscle fibres innervated by it. All fibres respond together. The number of fibres per neuron determines the degree of control. For example, in hands, there are only few muscle fibres per neuron. This gives very fine control and precise movement of the digits. The degree of control required in a large muscle group like the quadriceps is much less therefore each neuron innervates a large number of muscle fibres (Figure 2.4).

Types of muscle fibres

Muscle fibres are divided into two groups: Type 1 and Type 2

Type I Fibres. These are sometimes known as slow-twitch muscle fibres. Slow twitch refers to how often the neurons innervating the muscle fire to keep the muscle working. These muscles obtain their energy by aerobic respiration and are muscle groups that do prolonged/low-intensity work. These are the muscles of posture

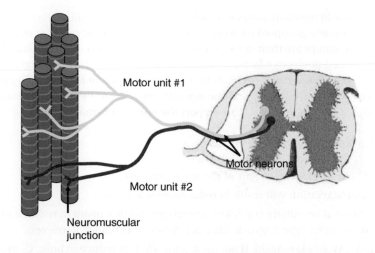

Figure 2.4   Motor unit consists of a single neuron and all the muscle fibres innervated by it. Akers and Denbow Anatomy and Physiology of Domestic Animals. Figure 7.16. Reproduced with permission of Wiley.

and core stability. This work is primarily seen in the postural muscle. They would include the paraspinal groups, and the internal and external abdominal obliques. Type I fibres are also found in the quadriceps and triceps along with type II fibres.

Type II Fibres. These are often referred to as fast-twitch muscles as the innervating neurons fire more often than their slow-twitch counterparts.

Type II fibres are further divided into Type IIa and Type IIb fibres. Type IIa are the long-distance muscles that are used for stamina and endurance, and use aerobic respiration. Type IIb are the speed muscles used in short bursts, and use anaerobic respiration.

Often type IIb muscles are plump round muscles such as the acromion head of deltoid. By contrast, the spinous head of deltoid is more strap-like, typical of a type IIa muscle.

Breed differences and training

Breeds such as huskies are bred for endurance and will have more type IIa fibres. Border collies will have a mixture of type IIa and type IIb fibres. Breeds such as whippets will have more type IIb fibres.

Training regimes can affect the predominance of one or other type of fibre. For instance, long-distance training with the dog running for great lengths of time at a steady pace will promote type IIa fibres. Interval training, where the dog does a short sprint for 1 minute followed by a walk for 2 minutes repeated over the course of 20 minutes will promote type IIb fibres.

Immobilisation

Immobilisation or prolonged inactivity, for example, cage rest, leads to atrophy of type I fibres first, followed by disuse atrophy of type II fibres. Where there has been loss of type I fibres, core stability will be significantly affected. If there is disuse atrophy of muscle that would normally support a joint, then often there will be recruitment of neighbouring muscle groups to try to stabilise the joint and these may not be postural muscles. These groups are then not available for locomotion and often become chronically tight or tied down to adjoining muscle groups and fascia. An example of this would be deep and superficial pectorals becoming tied down in long-standing shoulder problems where the supra- and infraspinatii muscles and subscapularis muscle have atrophied and no longer able to support the joint in normal posture.

Factors affecting muscle mass

Age. Muscle mass decreases as part of the ageing process.

Diet. Poor diet/starvation will result in reduced muscle mass.

Hereditary. Several hereditary conditions are recognised that result in reduced muscle mass, for example, type 2 muscle fibre deficiency in Labrador Retrievers.

Disuse atrophy. Wolff's law again. If not used, a muscle will reduce in bulk. Conversely training can increase muscle bulk.

Wallerian degeneration. A lower motor neuron lesion (LMN) will significantly reduce muscle mass very quickly.

Endocrine diseases. Diseases such as Cushing's disease, diabetes mellitus and hypothyroidism will also result in reduced muscle mass and muscle tone.

Types of contraction
Isometric
An isometric contraction is a muscle contraction but with no joint movement. An example of this would be a dog playing with a tug toy. This is something to bear in mind when drawing up a home exercise programme where joint movement may be painful or produce unwanted wear on a joint. In this situation, increasing muscle bulk may be desirable but not at the expense of further joint damage.

Isotonic
With an isotonic contraction, there is a joint movement when the muscle contracts.

There are two types of isotonic contraction: Concentric and Eccentric.

With a *Concentric* contraction, there is a shortening of muscle, for example, picking up shopping and bending the elbow.

With an *Eccentric* contraction, there is lengthening of muscle fibres, for example, lowering the shopping basket by extending the elbow.

Why is this important?
In general, eccentric contractions build muscles quicker. An eccentric contraction followed by a concentric contraction is called plyometrics and is a very good way of building muscle in the *canine athlete* (see Chapter 8).

Contraction versus contracture
A contraction is a normal shortening of a muscle. It is under voluntary or involuntary control and is reversible.

A contracture is a fixed shortening of muscle and is pathological.

Skeleton

This is divided into axial (head, spine, ribs and sternum) and appendicular (legs) parts. The anatomy of the head will not be dealt with in this textbook.

Spine

The spinal column is made up of a series of vertebrae, most of which have a similar structure. Salient features of individual vertebrae that can be identified in the live dog will be highlighted. Most vertebrae (Figure 2.5) consist of a central neural canal, body, arch, dorsal spinous process, two transverse processes and two cranially pointing and two caudally pointing articular processes making up the facet joints with the vertebra cranially and caudally, respectively. The intervertebral discs are located between the bodies of the vertebrae.

The canine spine is divided into five regions. (Figure 2.6) The cervical (C) region consisting of 7 vertebrae, the thoracic (T) region consisting of 13 vertebrae, the lumbar (L) region consisting of 7 vertebrae, the sacral (S) region consisting of 3 fused vertebrae and the coccygeal (Co) region consisting of approximately 5–20 bones depending on the breed. Each vertebra is a number with a prefix identifying its location. There are 13 pairs of ribs and 8 sternebrae making up the breastbone or sternum.

Cervical spine

The atlas (C1) differs in shape from the other vertebrae. It has no dorsal spinous process but has two large wings that can be palpated just caudal to the skull. The axis (C2) has a prominent spinous process. The spinous processes of C3–C7 initially point cranially but become more vertical. The length of the spinous processes also increases in length.

The transverse processes of C6 are very large and can be palpated cranial to the thoracic inlet. Just caudal to these transverse processes is the C6–C7 disc space that can be carefully palpated by gently displacing the trachea from the midline.

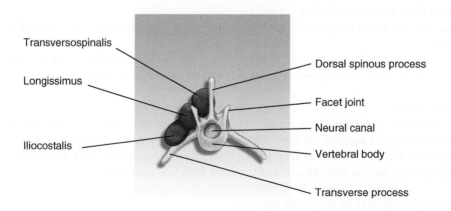

Transversospinalis

Longissimus

Iliocostalis

Dorsal spinous process

Facet joint

Neural canal

Vertebral body

Transverse process

Figure 2.5   Schematic representation of a vertebra head on showing body, neural canal, dorsal spinous process and transverse processes.

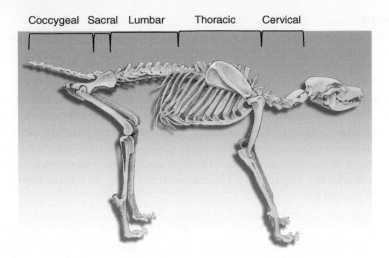

Coccygeal Sacral Lumbar   Thoracic   Cervical

Figure 2.6 Schematic drawing showing location of the cervical, thoracic, lumbar, sacral and coccygeal spine.

Thoracic spine
The thoracic vertebrae, T1–T11, have long spinous processes that point caudally initially but gradually become more vertical and shorter. T11 is referred to as the 'anticlinal' vertebra as the spinous process is perpendicular. The spinous processes of T12–13 point cranially. The thoracic vertebrae have an articulation with the ribs on each side. The first nine pairs of ribs also articulate with the sternum. Each rib has a dorsal bony and ventral cartilage part jointed together by the costochondral junction.

Lumbar spine
The spinous processes point slightly cranially. The spinous process of L7 is very short and can be identified directly between the wings of the ilium.

Sacral and coccygeal spine
Sacrum consists of three fused vertebrae. It articulates with the ilium via the sacroiliac joint.

The coccygeal spine consists of up to 20 vertebrae making up the tail region. The dura mater of the meninges continues down as far as Co8 or further in most dogs.

Facet joints
In the neck, the facet joints are arranged horizontally affording easy lateral head movement. The angle of the facet joints becomes more vertical progressing down the spine so that by the lumbar area, the facet joints are now nearly vertical to accommodate the flexion and extension of the spine seen when running.

Bony landmarks of the front leg

Scapula. Palpable landmarks in the live dog are dorsal border, spine, acromion and supraglenoid tubercle from which the biceps brachii muscle originates (Figure 2.7).

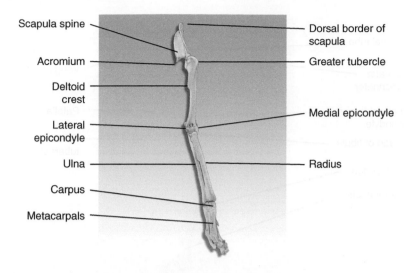

Scapula spine

Dorsal border of scapula

Acromium

Greater tubercle

Deltoid crest

Medial epicondyle

Lateral epicondyle

Ulna

Radius

Carpus

Metacarpals

Figure 2.7 Schematic drawing showing the bony landmarks of the front leg including scapula, humerus, radius, ulna, carpus and foot.

Humerus. Palpable bony landmarks, greater and lesser tubercle, bicipital groove, transverse ligament, deltoid tuberosity and lateral and medial epicondyle.

Radius and Ulna. Bony landmarks, radial head and styloid process. Ulna Olecranon, anconeal process, trochlear notch, medial and lateral coronoid processes and styloid process.

Carpus and front leg. Bony landmarks, Radial carpal bone, ulna carpal bone, accessory carpal bone, numbered carpal bones, five metacarpals, digits. Fifth metacarpophalangeal joint. Digit 1 has two phalanges, digits 2–5 have three.

Bony landmarks of the back leg

Pelvis. Formed from, ilium, ischium and pubis. Bony landmarks, dorsal spine of ilium, ischial tuberosity, obturator foramen and acetabulum.

Femur. Bony landmarks, head, greater trochanter, second trochanter, medial and lateral condyles, trochlear groove, patella and fabellae.

Tibia and fibular. Bony landmarks, tibial plateau, tibial tuberosity, medial malleolus, fibular head, body and lateral malleolus.

Tarsus and back foot. Calcaneus, talus, central, fourth tarsal bone. Fifth metatarsalphalangeal joint. Digit 1 may be missing. Digits 2–5 have three phalanges (Figure 2.8).

Shoulder joint
The shoulder joint is described as a ball-and-socket joint with the glenoid of the scapula forming the socket and the humeral head forming the body. However, the humeral head is far larger than the glenoid and the joint has been compared to a soccer ball sitting on a saucer. The joint capsule has thickenings medially and laterally

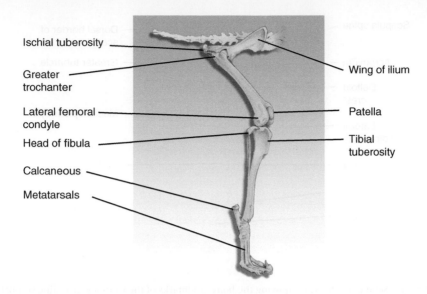

Ischial tuberosity

Greater trochanter

Lateral femoral condyle

Head of fibula

Calcaneous

Metatarsals

Wing of ilium

Patella

Tibial tuberosity

Figure 2.8 Schematic drawing showing the bony landmarks of the back leg, including the pelvis, femur, tibia, fibular, hock and foot.

making up the medial and lateral glenohumeral ligaments, respectively. In humans, there is a large rotator cuff around the joint that helps prevent dislocation when throwing. In dogs, there is no rotator cuff (usually) and the joint is dependent on the tone and strength of its intrinsic muscles for stability. In the dog the shoulder is a weight-bearing joint (Figure 2.9).

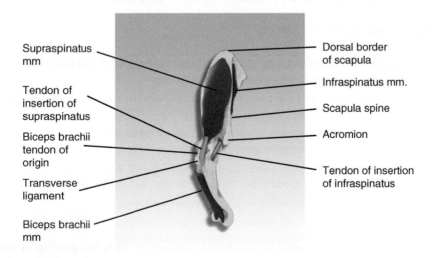

Supraspinatus mm

Tendon of insertion of supraspinatus

Biceps brachii tendon of origin

Transverse ligament

Biceps brachii mm

Dorsal border of scapula

Infraspinatus mm.

Scapula spine

Acromion

Tendon of insertion of infraspinatus

Figure 2.9 Schematic drawing of the shoulder cuff of the dog.

Important muscles in the shoulder

Subscapularis covers the medial aspect of the scapula and inserts onto medial humeral head. It provides medial support for the joint.

Supraspinatus originates from the supraspinatus fossa, the area on the scapula cranial to the spine, and inserts cranially onto greater tubercle. Its tendon of insertion runs close to the tendon of origin of biceps brachii and in pathological conditions can impinge on the biceps tendon. Supraspinatus extends and stabilises the shoulder joint.

Infraspinatus originates from the infraspinatus fossa, the area on the scapula caudal to the spine, and inserts on the lateral aspect of the greater tubercle. Its action is to flex or extend the shoulder depending upon position, abduct and outwardly rotate the joint as well as acting as a joint stabiliser.

Biceps brachii (Figure 2.10) originates from the supraglenoid tubercle of the scapula. Its origin is within the shoulder joint itself. Despite its name, the muscle only has one belly but does bifurcate distally to insert onto radial head and coronoid process of ulna. Its actions are to extend the shoulder *and* flex the elbow. This muscle crosses both the shoulder and elbow. It is innervated by the musculocutaneous nerve.

Triceps brachii (Figure 2.11). Despite its name, triceps brachii in the dog has four heads. Three heads, medial, accessory and lateral, originate from proximal humerus (medially, caudally and laterally, respectively) and insert onto the olecranon. Their action is to extend the elbow. The long head of triceps originates from caudal border of scapula and also inserts onto the olecranon. Its actions are to extend the elbow *and* flex the shoulder. Long head of triceps crosses two joints. It forms the main bulk in the caudal arm and is the main antigravity muscle in the front leg. All four heads are innervated by the radial nerve.

Pectoral girdle

The front leg of the dog is attached to the body by a muscle sling. The sling is made up of ventral serratus muscle that originates from the transverse processes of the last

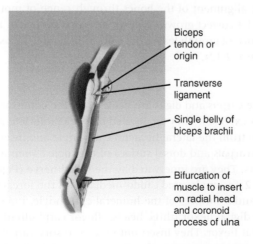

Biceps tendon or origin

Transverse ligament

Single belly of biceps brachii

Bifurcation of muscle to insert on radial head and coronoid process of ulna

Figure 2.10 Schematic drawing of the origin, course and insertion of the biceps brachii muscle.

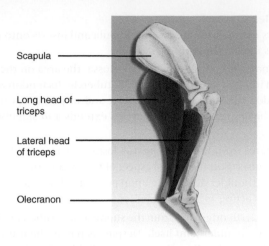

Scapula

Long head of triceps

Lateral head of triceps

Olecranon

Figure 2.11   Schematic drawing of the origin and insertion of the triceps group of muscles.

five cervical vertebrae and the first seven ribs and inserts on to dorsal third of the medial scapula. Its action is to support the trunk and depress the scapula.

The pectoral muscles (deep and superficial) originate from the sternum and insert onto the humeral tubercles. The deep pectoral bifurcates at its insertion around the tendon of origin of biceps brachii. The action of the pectorals is to draw the trunk cranially when the front leg is advanced when weight bearing or to draw the leg caudally when not weight bearing, and they also flex the shoulder.

Other muscles acting on the front leg are latissimus dorsi, a digging muscle, and trapezius, which elevates and abducts the leg.

Elbow joint
The elbow is an inherently stable joint, unlike the shoulder. It has true ligaments to maintain correct alignment of the bones through range of motion. The elbow is a complex joint and a correct growth synergy between humerus, radius and ulna is vital. This fine balance of growth leaves the elbow vulnerable to a series of pathological conditions (Figure 2.12).

Extensors
The extensors of the carpus and digits are made up of the extensor carpi radialis and the common digital extensor. They are located on the cranio-lateral part of the forearm. They originate from the lateral humeral epicondyle and insert onto the cranial surface of the metacarpals and dorsal surface of the digits. Their action is to extend the carpus and digits. They are innervated by the radial nerve (Figure 2.13).

Flexors (Figure 2.14) are located caudo-medially on the forearm. They originate from medial and caudal surfaces of the humeral epicondyle, radius and ulna. They consist of the deep digital flexor (three heads,) flexor carpi ulnaris (two heads) and the superficial digital flexor. They insert onto the accessory carpal bone and palmer surface of the digits. Their action is to flex the carpus and digits. They are innervated by the median and ulnar nerves.

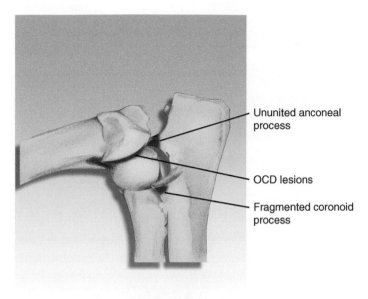

Ununited anconeal
process

OCD lesions

Fragmented coronoid
process

Figure 2.12 Schematic drawing of an elbow joint opened up to demonstrate where the various pathologies occur.

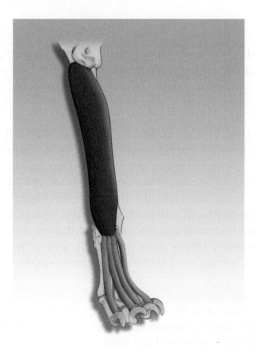

Figure 2.13 Schematic drawing of the extensor group of muscles that are located craniolaterally on the forearm.

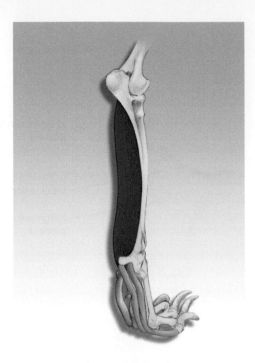

Figure 2.14   Schematic drawing of the flexor group of muscles that are located caudo-medially on the forearm.

Hip
The hip joint is a rigid ball-and-socket joint. Stability is further increased by the labrum and joint capsule, round ligament and the large muscle mass surrounding the joint.

Gluteals
This muscle mass consists of deep, middle and superficial gluteal. This group of muscles originates from ilium, ischial spine, sacrum and sacrotuberous ligament. They all insert on greater trochanter or just distal on third trochanter. Their action is to extend the hip. They also have some involvement in internal rotation of the hip and abduction of the leg. Innervation is by the gluteal nerves (Figure 2.15).

The piriformis muscle is fused with the middle gluteal muscle except in carnivores. It runs from the lateral side of the caudal sacral and first coccygeal vertebrae to the greater trochanter, where it inserts along with middle gluteal. Its action is to extend and abduct the hip. It is innervated by the caudal gluteal nerve.

Quadriceps
The quadriceps mass occupies the cranio-medial, cranial and cranio-lateral thigh. The group inserts onto tibial tuberosity via a large tendon incorporating the patella. The action of the group is to extend the stifle. Certain parts of the group (rectus femoris and cranial sartorius) also flex the hip. Innervation is by the femoral nerve (Figure 2.16).

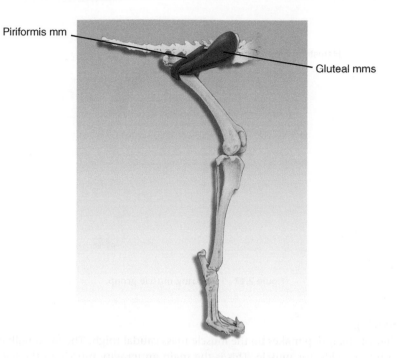

Piriformis mm

Gluteal mms

Figure 2.15   Gluteal muscle group.

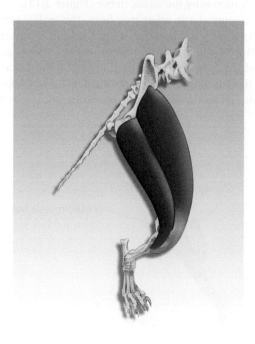

Figure 2.16   Quadriceps muscle group.

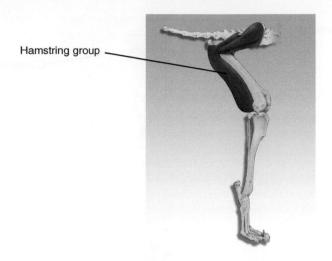

Figure 2.17   Hamstring muscle group.

Hamstrings

The hamstring group makes up the muscle mass caudal thigh. The main bulk is provided by the adductor muscle. This is the main antigravity muscle in the back leg. The main actions of the hamstrings are to flex the stifle and extend the hip. They also adduct the leg. Innervation is by the sciatic nerve (Figure 2.17).

Gracilis muscle (Figure 2.18) originates from the pubic symphysis. It has a cylindrical muscle belly but ends in a very long tendon that inserts on the cranial border of the tibia. The tendon of insertion also attaches to the crural fascia that runs down to form part of the Achilles tendon that inserts on the calcaneus. This muscle can be palpated in the live dog in the caudo-medial thigh. It extends the hip and adducts the leg. It also flexes the stifle and extends the hock. It is innervated by the obturator nerve.

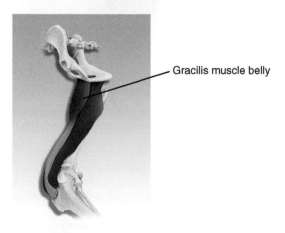

Figure 2.18   Gracilis mm.

The pectineus muscle is a cigar-shaped muscle with a long tendon of insertion that runs in the groin. It originates from the pubis and inserts onto medial condyle of femur. Its action is to adduct the leg. This muscle can usually be easily identified close to the femoral artery and vein. Often with hip issues this muscle is tight. It is innervated by the obturator nerve.

The stifle consists of two joints: the femoro-patella joint and the femoro-tibial joint. The femoro-patella joint consists of the trochlear groove in which the patella (a sesamoid in the quadriceps tendon of insertion) runs. There are medial and lateral patellar ligaments, but these can be quite discreet and are part of the medial and lateral retinaculae.

In the femoro-tibial joint, the femoral condyles sit on the tibial plateau. The medial and lateral menisci sit between the two bones. The menisci are made of fibrocartilage and act as shock absorbers. They are held in place by meniscotibial ligaments. The stifle joint has a medial and lateral collateral ligament and a cranial and caudal cruciate ligament.

Cruciate ligaments

In the centre of the joint are the cruciate ligaments. The cranial cruciate ligament originates from the caudomedial surface of the lateral femoral condyle and inserts on the cranial intercondylar area of the tibia. It passes cranial to the caudal cruciate ligament that originates from the lateral side of the medial femoral condyle and inserts on the caudal aspect of the tibia. (Figure 2.19) The cranial cruciate ligament is made up of two bands: the cranio-medial band and the caudo-lateral band. The cranio-medial band accounts for only about 15% of the CCL. It is taut in flexion and loose in extension. The caudo-lateral band makes up the remaining 85%. It is loose in flexion and taut in extension. Partial tears usually occur to the cranio-medial band.

Two fabellae are located caudal to each femoral condyle. These are sesamoids in the tendons of origin of the gastrocnemius muscles.

The main action of the stifle is flexion and extension. Rotation is limited.

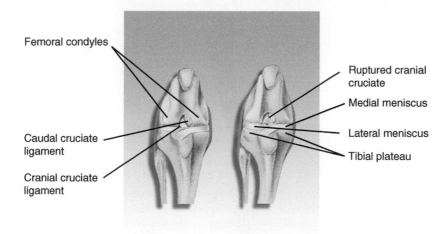

Figure 2.19 Cruciate ligaments.

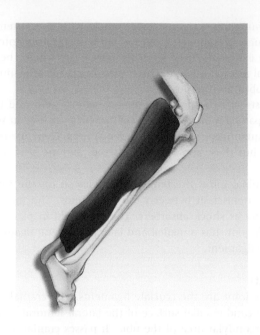

Figure 2.20   Gastrocnemicus mm.

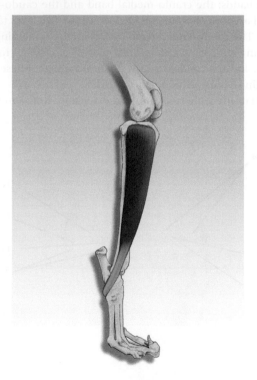

Figure 2.21   Cranial tibial mm.

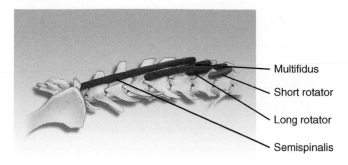

Multifidus

Short rotator

Long rotator

Semispinalis

Figure 2.22   Multifidus mm.

Gastrocnemius muscles (Figure 2.20) originate from the medial and lateral supra-condylar tuberosities of the femur. They insert onto calcaneus. Their action is to flex the stifle and extend the tarsus. Innervation is by the tibial branch of the sciatic nerve.

The Achilles tendon is composed of the common tendon of insertion of the gas-trocnemius muscles insert onto calcaneus. The crural fascia also inserts at this point. Part of the tendon of the superficial digital flexor also inserts onto calcaneus. How-ever, the remainder of the superficial digital flexor tendon runs over the point of calcaneus (in a small groove) and inserts onto the planter surface of the digits. Note that the superficial digital flexor muscle originates *deep* to the gastrocnemius muscles and the tendons twist around each other at the proximal edge of the Achilles tendon.

Cranial tibia muscle (Figure 2.21) originates from the lateral side of the cranial tibia and inserts onto the planter surface of the first two metatarsal. Its actions are to flex the tarsus and to supinate the paw. Innervation is by the tibial branch of the sciatic nerve.

Muscles of the trunk
Included in this group are the internal and external abdominal obliques and the rectus abdominus that form the belly. Other trunk muscles are trapezius, latissimus dorsi and omotransversarius and the paraspinals.

The paraspinal muscles are arranged in three layers (Figures 2.5 and 2.22).

The transversospinalis, the longissimus and the iliocostalis groups.

Layers of paraspinal muscles: The transversospinalis mm all originate from the spinous process of a cranial vertebra and insert on mammillary processes of the facet joint a specified number of vertebrae caudal to the vertebra of origin.

Transversospinalis: Action: Rotate the vertebrae.

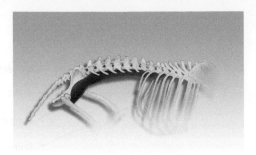

Figure 2.23   Iliopsoas mm.

Short Rotator 1 vertebra; Long Rotator 2 vertebrae; Semispinalis 5 vertebrae and *Multifidus* 3 vertebrae – Multifidus mm are PROPRIOCEPTIVE rather than motor and are very important feedback muscles for posture, core stability and proprioception.

Longissimus mm rotate, extend and laterally flex the thoracic and lumbar spine.

Iliocostalis laterally flexes the lumbar spine.

Iliopsoas (Figure 2.23). In a cow, this constitutes the fillet steak cut or Chateaubriand for the whole muscle. It originates from the ventral surface of transverse processes of T9-L7 vertebrae and the ventral border of ilium. It inserts onto second trochanter of femur. This is the muscle that often leaves a little tag when doing an FHO. It is important to preserve this muscle. Its actions are to flex and outwardly rotate the hip and flex the lumbar spine. The femoral nerve that passes through the muscle innervates it. This muscle is commonly injured.

CHAPTER 3

Healing

When the body sustains an injury there are two ways it can heal the wound: repair and regeneration. This chapter is mainly concerned with and covers the processes involved in the repair of soft tissues. Following an injury, the body goes through a consistent and organised healing process, which involves a series of events. It is generally agreed that there are four stages, but some authors do include injury as a separate event. These stages are inflammation, proliferation, repair and remodelling. Even though they are often thought of as four separate stages, they actually overlap heavily and should be thought as a continuum of activity that is dependent on one stage occurring to initiate progression to the next stage. The progression to each stage depends on the chemical and cellular processes that occur and the healing tissue's ability to respond to specific stresses placed on it (Figure 3.1).

This chapter is mainly concerned with describing events in the healing process after an injury. However, this process can also be initiated by other events such as repetitive microtrauma, mechanical irritation, excessive heating or cooling, infection and autoimmune diseases. We cannot normally accelerate the healing process, but by having knowledge of the healing process, we can advise clients on how to avoid poor and delayed healing.

Stages of healing

Inflammation

Inflammation is the body's natural response to an injury and it needs to occur to begin the complex process of healing. In the inflammatory stage, the body reacts to the injury by stimulating the clearance of the area of any debris, infection and dead cells in order to prepare it for the repair. During this phase, the cells that clear the damaged area and begin the formation of scar tissue are brought to the area in the tissue fluid or inflammatory exudate. The inflammatory response begins within an hour of the injury, but reaches full effect 1–2 days after the injury, on average. More vascular tissues will reach their peak quicker.

The amount of inflammation is directly related to the amount of trauma sustained. A major injury will pass through acute, subacute and chronic phases of inflammation. The inflammatory stage has vascular and cellular events that occur simultaneously and are heavily interlinked.

Practical Physiotherapy for Small Animal Practice, First Edition.
Edited by David Prydie and Isobel Hewitt.
© 2015 John Wiley & Sons, Ltd. Published 2015 by John Wiley & Sons, Ltd.
Companion Website: www.wiley.com/go/practical-physiotherapy-for-small-animals

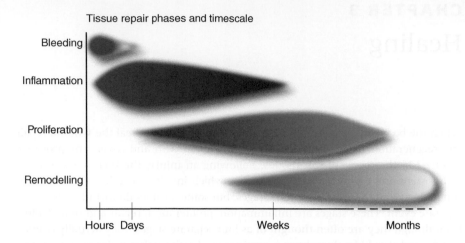

Tissue repair phases and timescale

Bleeding

Inflammation

Proliferation

Remodelling

Hours Days   Weeks   Months

Figure 3.1   *Timescale of healing.* The healing stages occur successively and overlap over days, months and years.

There are four cardinal signs of injury: *Pain (dolor), swelling (tubor), redness (rubor) and heat (calor).*

Pain occurs as a result of mechanical and chemical influences.

Swelling occurs as a result of the vascular response to injury and the outpouring of tissue fluid.

Redness is also a result of the vascular response due to the increase in local blood flow.

Heat is produced again by the increase in blood flow and chemical mediators.

Initially, the tissue haemorrhages as blood vessel walls are damaged and transient vasoconstriction initiated by the release of noradrenaline (norepinephrine) is followed by vasodilation. The intact blood vessels near the wound site also experience changes. There is an increase in blood flow, and dormant capillary beds can be opened to increase blood flow into the wounded area. The amount of bleeding is dependent on the type of tissue damaged and the extent of the injury. Damage to the blood vessels means cells beyond the area of damage will not receive sufficient oxygen and they will subsequently die. Damage to the tissues initiates the release of chemical mediators and attracts cells such as mast cells to the area.

Mast cells release histamine, which increases vasodilation, and they also start forming a jelly-like scar tissue. Bradykinins are released by the dead cells. This increases the permeability of the blood vessel walls allowing blood, plasma and cells to leak into the tissues. The bradykinins have other important actions during the inflammatory stage, such as activation of substance P and enhancement of the release of prostaglandins. Prostaglandins increase vasodilation and their effect lasts longer than that of histamine. Substance P will also promote vasodilation and increase vascular permeability. The dead cells, tissue fluid and blood fill the area. Tissue bleeding needs to be arrested as soon as possible as the blood will act as an irritant, increasing pain and prolonging the inflammatory process.

Blood loss stimulates platelet activity, which will initiate coagulation by releasing phospholipids, and thus the formation of a clot. Platelet plugs are formed in the presence of thrombin, which is released by the platelets themselves to stimulate platelet aggregation and adhesion. At this time, the lymphatic system is also plugged to limit the amount of tissue fluid leaking into the damaged area. The coagulation of the tissue fluid and platelet plugs adheres to tissue walls and provides a wound matrix that can attract further cells to the area.

The immature clot is further strengthened by strands of fibrin that are deposited in the clot by fibronectin (a structural glycoprotein), which is like tissue 'glue' and other adhesive proteins such as fibrinogen and thrombospondin. This 'glue' provides the tensile strength for the wound during the inflammatory stage and it helps to trap debris/foreign material in preparation for the white blood cells to remove them. The wound matrix/clot acts as an early scar and becomes a scaffold for development of the scar in the proliferation stage. The platelets also release growth factors that will stimulate angiogenesis and help control fibrin deposition in the proliferation phase (Figure 3.2).

Chemical and mechanical stimuli, such as the presence of bacteria, cell factors and chemical mediators (substance P, prostaglandin and histamine), act as attractants to the white blood cells – monocytes, macrophages, leukocytes and neutrophils. Monocytes are cells that can differentiate into other cells and in this environment, they will as act macrophages. The job of macrophages, leukocytes and neutrophils is to clear the wound environment by phagocytosis to provide a sound foundation for the repair. The macrophages release digestive enzymes, collagenase and proteoglycan, to remove the necrotic tissue, foreign material, debris, bacteria and dying neutrophils. Lactic acid is produced during phagocytosis and it acts as a stimulant for the proliferation phase. The macrophages will also direct the repair process by releasing chemical factors that attract and activate the fibroblastic repair cells, which are the major cells involved in the formation of scar tissue in the proliferation phase (Figure 3.3).

Pain in the inflammatory stage can be caused by mechanical and chemical influences. Mechanical pain arises from the actual tissue damage, neurological reflex inhibition, protective muscle spasm (which occurs to prevent movement of the injured area) and pressure of the tissue oedema on the surrounding tissues. Chemical pain is caused when the nerve receptors (or nociceptors) in the injured area are activated and sensitised by chemicals, such as bradykinins, prostaglandins and histamine. If the pain stimulus prolongs, then the nociceptors can be overstimulated or irritated by the chemicals causing high levels of pain, although there is no actual damage occurring at the nerve endings. This may lead to a state of hyperalgesia (see Chapter 10), and it is thought that the prostaglandins are responsible for sensitising the nociceptors which increases their response to painful stimuli.

Proliferation

This stage starts when the scar is formed and the repair process begins. This begins 24–48 hours after injury and its peak response occurs after 2–3 weeks.

The fibroblasts attracted to the wound site by macrophages in the inflammatory stage will start to make collagen, which is the basic building block of scar tissue.

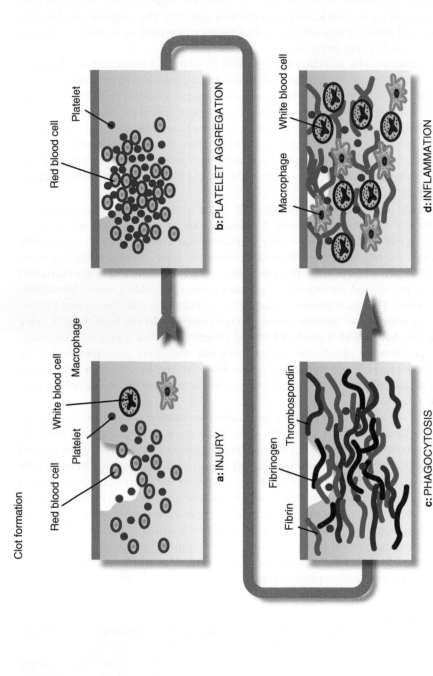

Figure 3.2 *Clot formation.* Coagulation of the blood starts the formation of a clot that is further strengthened by fibrin, fibrinogen and thrombospondin.

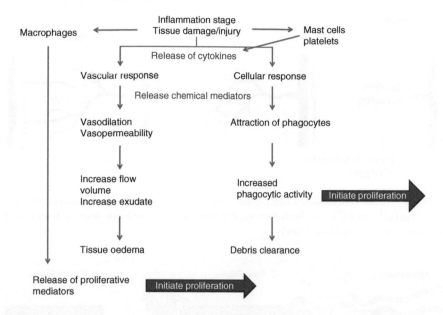

Figure 3.3 *Inflammation.* The inflammatory stage has a series of chemical mediators that are released to stimulate the continuation of the inflammatory stage and initiate the proliferation stage.

The fibroblasts take over from the macrophages as the director cell in the proliferation phase and increase in number until they reach a maximal number, 5–10 days after the injury.

The production of collagen requires oxygen. In the injury, damage to blood vessels interrupts the blood supply thus leaving a hypoxic environment. The early proliferation stage is concerned with forming a vascular bed of new blood vessels; this process is called angiogenesis.

Angiogenesis overlaps the inflammation and proliferation stages with the early capillaries beginning to develop 12 hours after injury and the process continuing over the next 2–3 days. It is vital for the proliferation stage to provide enough oxygen, cell migration and nutrition to the wound site for repair to take place. These new blood vessels are fragile and can be easily damaged. Angiogenesis is stimulated by multiple factors and it starts with capillary buds sprouting. The capillary buds grow towards areas where there are low concentrations of oxygen. These buds attract endothelial cells to attach to them and the buds increase in size, thereby forming loops. Further buds are formed from these loops, thus creating a network of vessels. These vessels develop lumina within themselves, and anastomosis occurs in existing vessels, which then establishes a blood flow (Figure 3.4).

Fibronectin found in the wound area in the inflammatory stage acts a chemical attractant to fibroblasts, facilitates their attachment to fibrin and increases the migration of further fibroblasts to the area. The fibroblasts have multiple roles in the proliferation phase: to secrete a ground substance, produce collagen and some differentiate into myofibroblasts. To produce collagen, the fibroblasts create tropocollagen molecules that are singular and do not have any cross links. The ground substance will

Angiogenesis

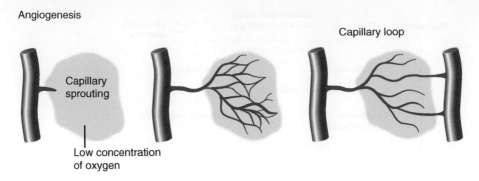

Capillary loop

Capillary sprouting

Low concentration of oxygen

Figure 3.4 *Capillary bed formation.* The capillary buds sprout and grow towards areas of hypoxia. Endothelial cells attach to the buds forming capillary loops. These loops develop lumina and anastomosis to existing blood vessels.

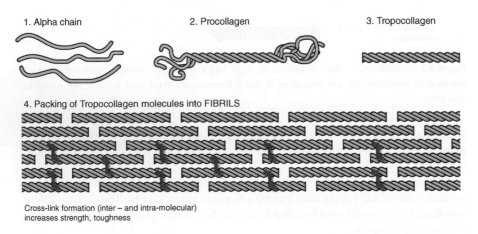

1. Alpha chain

2. Procollagen

3. Tropocollagen

4. Packing of Tropocollagen molecules into FIBRILS

Cross-link formation (inter – and intra-molecular) increases strength, toughness

Figure 3.5 *Formation of collagen fibrils.* Fibrils are formed by molecules of tropocollagen bunching together and developing cross links.

provide a cross-linking mechanism for the tropocollagen molecules that can 'glue' the wound together and the myofibroblasts have a contractile action, which will help to seal the wound. The cross links between the tropocollagen molecules mean they bunch together into fibrils. The fibrils will polymerise into bundles of collagen (Figure 3.5). The collagen produced at this early stage is usually type 3, but type 1 is also produced. As the scar matures in the presence of hyaluronic acid, and as fibrinogen is reduced, type 1 becomes the predominant tissue.

The different types of collagen have slightly different properties:

Type 1 is found in mature scar tissue as it has good ability to withstand tension.

Type 2 can withstand pressure.

Type 3 is the main type found during healing as it does not have the ability to withstand great tension or pressure due to its thin, weak fibres.

As the scar develops and matures, it will also develop nerve receptors that are sensitive to tension and pressure. The collagen that initially formed and 'laid down' is haphazard and the nerve receptors will signal where the lines of stress are within the tissue, allowing collagen to orientate itself along these.

As collagen is formed, it shortens. Therefore, collagen fibres in a small wound are enough to bind the edges of the wound together and provide enough tensile strength to withstand normal movement in approximately 7 days; however, if the wound is larger, granulation tissue is formed as well and it can be several weeks before enough collagen is laid down to provide the tensile strength to withstand normal movement. In larger wounds, contraction occurs via myofibroblasts. These contract to draw the wound edges together, thus reducing the wound size. This is thought to occur as the myofibroblasts attach themselves to the collagen fibres and contract, holding the collagen in place until it stabilises.

As the granulation tissue increases in the wound site, the original fibrin clot decreases in size. As the fibrin clot is destroyed and the new collagen is being produced, the tensile strength is at its lowest level. The mechanism for the metabolism and production of collagen is regulated by cytokines, which balance the release of collagenase to remove the fibrin clot and stimulation of new collagen being produced.

The formation and alignment of collagen is initially random and the number of fibres laid down increases substantially in the first 3 weeks after the injury. During this time, the tensile strength of the injured area also increases not just because of the increase in the number of fibres but also as a result of the development of collagen cross links and the orientation of the fibres within the tissue. The scar tissue will achieve approximately 15–20% of its tensile strength in the first 3 weeks of formation (Figure 3.6).

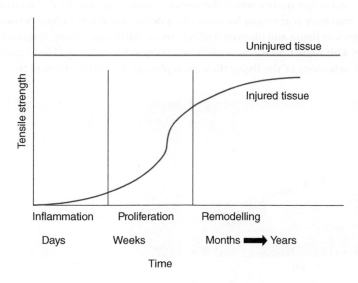

Figure 3.6 *Tensile strength of collagen.* Following injury, the tensile strength increases slowly in the inflammatory stage and then rapidly in the proliferation stage. The tensile strength will remain slightly less than the uninjured tissue.

The immature scar tissue initially appears red and swollen. This is due to an increase in fluid and the extensive vascular system. This scar is tender and is easily damaged by pressure and stretching. Towards the end of the proliferation stage and into the remodelling stage, the area begins to lose its vascularity and fluid, therefore the scar tissue starts to become more densely packed.

Repair or remodelling

This stage is where the scar formed in the proliferation stage is made into a functional repair. It begins approximately 1 week after the inflammatory stage fades out; however, most agree it begins in earnest from approximately 21 days and can continue for up to 2 years until a fully avascular scar replaces the immature gel-like scar tissue. This occurs as the capillaries regress and become ingested by macrophages. Other cellular components of the extracellular matrix also reduce, such as macrophages, fibroblasts and myofibroblasts. The scar tissue becomes whiter and will be less sensitive to pressure and tension (Figure 3.7(a) and (b)).

The new scar tissue formed will, during the remodelling stage, become more like the tissue it is replacing or in some tissues it is the regeneration of the tissue. The collagen in the scar tissue responds to the physical stresses put on it and lines itself up along these stress lines. The scar tissue will not have the same tensile strength or properties of the tissue it is replacing, but through remodelling it will come to closely resemble that tissue and enable restoration of normal function. The final structural arrangement of fibres and their orientation are due to the remodelling phase.

The arrangement and orientation of the fibres are random, following the proliferation phase and this immature, weak scar tissue begins to align the fibres along a lateral and linear orientation. The orientation of fibres occurs through tension and induction. Induction occurs when the normal tissue adjacent to the wound influences the immature scar tissue; for example, a dense tissue will induce dense heavily cross-linked scar tissue and likewise a pliable tissue will induce loose, less cross-linked scar tissue. This induction is responsible for collagen fibres being able to take on the functional behaviour of the tissue they are replacing. The orientation of the collagen

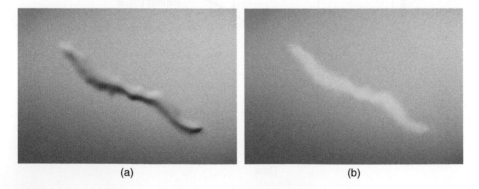

(a)   (b)

Figure 3.7 *Immature (a) and mature (b) scar tissue.* Immature scar tissue initially appears red and swollen. This is due to an increase in fluid and the extensive vascular system. Mature scar tissue begins to lose its vascularity and fluid, therefore the scar tissue starts to become more densely packed and becomes white in appearance.

Collagen orientation

Without tension = random orientation
of collagen = weakness

With tension = collagen oriented along
straight lines = strength

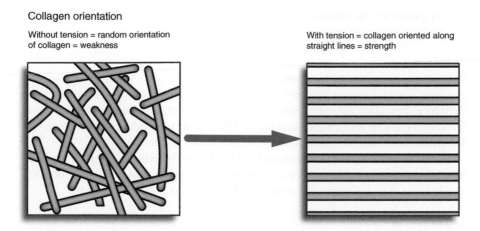

Figure 3.8   *Fibre orientation/lines of stress in collagen.* The arrangement and orientation of the fibres are random following the proliferation phase. The fibres begin to align along lateral and linear orientation.

fibres is also influenced by the internal and external stresses placed on the wound as they are remodelling. These stresses include joint movement, muscle tension, loading and unloading of connective tissue and mobilisation, which can strongly influence the fibre orientation, in effect physiotherapy. It is important that normal movement is encouraged at this stage so that the orientation of the fibres is along the correct directional pull. The collagen fibres contract and shorten as they mature. Therefore, the mobilisation of the scar is important to repeatedly stretch the collagen (Figure 3.8).

The cross-linking system within the collagen that is formed during the proliferation stage is a weak system that consists of hydrogen bonding; however, during the remodelling stage, these bonds are strengthened and become covalent bonds. The hydrogen bonds are relatively weak to allow the scar tissue to be gently mobilised. As the scar matures, the stronger covalent bonds do not yield to stress as easily, the cross links become more prolific and the tissue is more dense and resilient than the immature scar.

During the remodelling stage, the scar is reorganised as the fibres are reorientated, replaced and absorbed. It is important that an appropriate balance between collagen synthesis and reabsorption is found and stresses applied to the healing wound do not alter this one way or the other. The synthesis and reorganisation of the collagen enable the tissue to return to normal functional activity 6–12 months after the injury; however, dense connective tissue, such as fascia, can take much longer time to achieve its maximum tensile strength.

Different tissue responses to healing

The amount of inflammation and whole healing process is heavily affected by the blood supply to the injured tissue. The more vascular a tissue is, the faster it can heal as the chemical mediators/cells, oxygen and nutrients required for healing are more readily available. The inflammatory stage fades after 8–10 days in vascular tissue and the proliferation stage peaks at 10–14 days.

Tendon

In tendons, the inflammatory process will begin to fade after 3 weeks. Tendons are not very vascular tissues and their structures do not allow for a collection of fluid, therefore they often do not exhibit much swelling following injury. The scar tissue formed in tendons is orientated into parallel lines as this provides the maximum tensile strength but also maintains the gliding properties of a tendon.

Tendons are designed to withstand high loads. On the other hand, they are often injured not through a single traumatic event but are fatigued by repetitive submaximal loading, which disrupts the structure of the tendon fibres (Figure 3.9).

Ligaments

Ligaments are relatively avascular structures, which means that they do not show dramatic swelling following injury. The scar tissue formed in ligaments needs to be very strong as the ligaments need to withstand excessive joint movements. But, when this tension is removed, they have to be able to relax. To allow the movement of the joint, the scar tissue between a ligament and bone needs to be randomly orientated and loose.

Muscle

The contractile force of a muscle is reduced by inflammation. Even if this inflammation is not evident, it can still cause muscle dysfunction. This damage can occur in skeletal muscles as a result of inactivity. Inactivity of a skeletal muscle will cause muscular atrophy, loss of strength and an increase in connective tissue that will reduce the ability of the muscle to contract. A reduction of contractile force will also be seen as

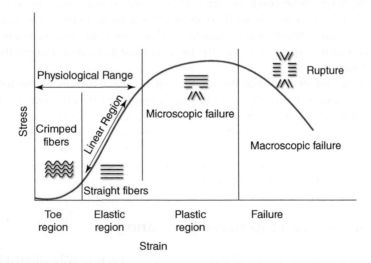

Figure 3.9 *Tendon injury/overloading.* Tendons can become injured following repetitive submaximal loading that will disrupt the structure of the tendon fibres.

a loss of strength. The scar tissue produced in a muscle belly needs to be very flexible and extensible to cope with the muscle contracting and stretching.

As muscles are vascular tissues, following injury, there can be considerable bleeding and swelling or haematoma formation.

Nerves

Following injury to a peripheral nerve, the damaged ends of the axon will seal themselves off and the axon distal to the wound site will begin to disintegrate. The endoneurium and neurolemma surrounding the axon remain intact. Schwann cells and macrophages will migrate into the area. The macrophages will phagocytise the axonal debris and the Schwann cells will proliferate and form cellular cords. These cords attach to the damaged ends of the axon and guide 'sprouts' to bridge the gap in the axon. The Schwann cells also remyelinate the regenerating axon and release growth factors to encourage axonal growth. The growth of a peripheral nerve can be 1–5 mm per day once the debris is cleared (this can take approximately a week), and hence the time it takes to heal is dependent on the size of the injury (Figure 3.10).

In the central nervous system, the nervous tissue will not regenerate if the damaged ends are farther than 1 mm apart; therefore, CNS damage is generally seen as irreversible. The functional recovery of the nervous system after trauma is seen because of neural re-training rather than healing of the neural tissue.

Bone

Bone is enclosed by periosteum, which contains osteoblasts (cells that forms new bone), and the bone cavity contains osteoclasts (bone-destroying cells). As in soft-tissue healing the first stage is when bleeding occurs and haematoma forms, osteogenic cells from the periosteum and medullary canal will proliferate and bridge the gap in the bone. Once the gap is bridged, osteoblasts and osteoclasts increase in numbers and new bone begins to be laid down, the repair is now called a callus and becomes more calcified as bone begins to bridge the gap. The osteoclasts will be working to clean up the area and remove dead bone. As the fracture site is stabilised by solid bone, remodelling begins with bone reabsorption removing excess bone, thickening of bone formed in areas of high stress and re-formation of the medullary canal. Studies have shown that the mechanical properties of bone alter depending on the level of stress placed on them. Resting a bone for a prolonged time (e.g. cage rest) will increase mineral reabsorption and therefore decrease the strength of the bone. It is important for bone to be placed under gentle stress as soon as the fracture site is stable to improve the quality of the bone formed (Figure 3.11).

Articular cartilage

Articular cartilage, as a structure, is designed to withstand high forces, however unexpected loading such as trauma does happen and tends to cause a slip or shear injury to the cartilage. An injury to the cartilage alone produces very poor healing as cartilage does not have a direct blood supply and usually gains its nutrition via osmosis from the synovial fluid of a joint. Some healing can occur with proliferation of fibroblasts invading from the local soft tissues. If the injury is more significant and the sub-chondral bone is damaged at the same time, then blood vessels can grow into the cartilage and healing occurs as described in the bone healing section.

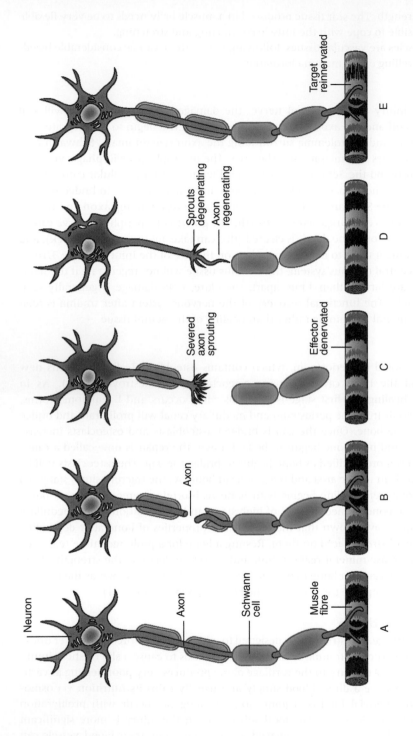

Figure 3.10 *Nerve regeneration/healing.* (a) normal neuron, (b) injury to neuron, (c) removal of damaged axon/debris and axonal sprouting, (d) regeneration and remyelination of axon and (e) re-innervation of muscle fibre.

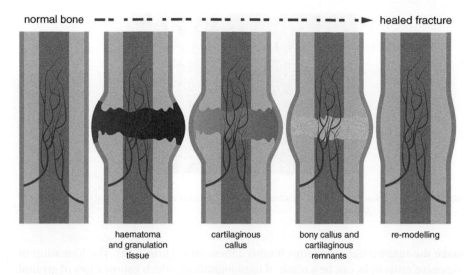

normal bone — — · — — · — — · — — · — — · — — ·▶ healed fracture

| haematoma and granulation tissue | cartilaginous callus | bony callus and cartilaginous remnants | re-modelling |

Figure 3.11 *Bone healing.* The healing of bone follows four stages: (a) haematoma formation, (b) callus formation, (c) callus hardening into solid bone and (d) bone remodelled.

The osteogenic cells from the periosteum can form fibrous tissue and fibrocartilage to heal the cartilage.

Consequences of maladaptive healing

Following an injury, the healing process is initiated, if at any point during the healing process another injury occurs to the tissue or they are overloaded, the healing process restarts. Repeated injuries will cause thickening of the scar tissue.

Inflammation stage

The inflammatory phase can be the start of maladaptive healing as in this stage very little inflammation will delay healing and will very much cause excessive scar tissue formation. Secondary inflammation following acute injury can occur when the healing breach is overstressed causing disruption of the early scar and stimulation of the body to produce more scar tissue, which can lead to adhesions and contractures. This will cause further pain, hamper the function of the soft tissue and start to cause a state of chronic inflammation, which will further deteriorate the function of the soft tissue. This can become difficult to treat as it is a self-perpetuating cycle.

The control of bleeding in the inflammatory phase is essential, as the formation of haematomas will disrupt wound healing by being a physical barrier to the approximation of the wound edges and the presence of a haematoma gives the ideal medium for infection. Infection of injured tissues is a serious complication as it increases the work of the white blood cells delaying the progression into the proliferation stage.

Proliferation stage

In the proliferation stage, the formation of cross links in the new scar tissue is responsible for its new tensile strength, but if the cross links become excessive, it will

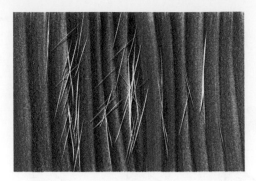

Figure 3.12   *Adhesion formation*. If the cross links become excessive, it will make the tissue tough and forms fibrous adhesions.

make the tissue tough and forms fibrous adhesions (Figure 3.12). The formation of excessive cross links can be a result of immobilisation, which causes a loss of ground substance. This will reduce the distance between the collagen fibres creating friction between the subunits.

The types of scars that are produced following abnormal healing are hypertrophic and keloid scars. Excessive collagen deposition in the original wound site is called hypertrophic scarring and excessive collagen in the tissues around the wound is called keloid scarring.

Also in the proliferation stage, contraction of the wound needs to be controlled as even a very little contraction can lead to excess bleeding and infection, which, as previously stated, can lead to further inflammation. Excessive contraction of the wound can lead to tissue contracture giving rise to deformity and dysfunction (Figure 3.13).

Even though this chapter is concerned with the healing process after a single injury, it is worth noting that many cases do arrive with overuse injuries. Overuse injuries or syndromes are where repetitive trauma from excessive movement or tension on weakened tissues disrupts the tissue unity and causes microtrauma.

These produce a chronic low-grade inflammation and it becomes very difficult to identify the onset of this type of injury. If the onset of injury is unknown, the stage of healing and amount of healing that has occurred already will be unknown. It is also more difficult to identify pain, swelling and lameness as they are often less evident. The chronic inflammation from an overuse injury may have been developing over weeks, months or even years, but can happen as a result of acute inflammation. They present quite a challenge for therapists to overcome but therapy can be very effective in dealing with these, since traditional rest and anti-inflammatory medicines have often failed. Overuse injuries are most commonly seen in working or sporting animals.

Factors that also affect healing

There are some other considerations as therapists/veterinarians need to consider when discussing the healing process such as age, medications and concurrent illnesses.

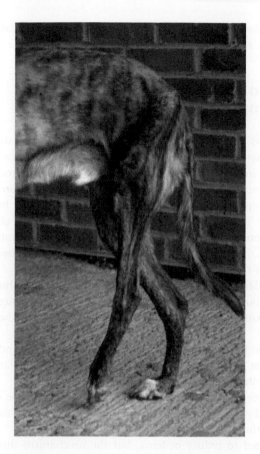

Figure 3.13 *Contracture.* Excessive contraction of the wound can lead to tissue contracture giving rise to deformity and dysfunction.

Age – As the body ages, the healing process slows. The migration and proliferation of cells are delayed along with wound contraction and collagen remodelling. Together, these can reduce the tensile strength of the new tissues which in turn leads to the wound being more likely to break down when stress is placed on it. There are also changes noted in the gel-fibre ratio that are similar to the changes noted when a joint or leg is immobilised. Therefore, as an animal ages, it is more likely to develop contractures.

Medications – Non-Steroidal Anti-Inflammatory drugs have different actions. Some do not alter the production of collagen and some do but they will inhibit production of histamine, serotonin and prostaglandins. The inhibition of prostaglandins will reduce oedema, reduce pain and allow the tissue to move into the proliferation stage. This will enable movement to occur without pain, enabling a quicker return to function.

Diabetes – Slows the healing process by affecting the inflammatory stage implying insulin has a role in the inflammatory process.

Temperature – Cellular activity decreases when temperature is reduced, which will delay healing.

Poor blood supply – Vascular insufficiency or ischaemia will delay healing by not allowing oxygen, cells, nutrition and chemical mediators to get to the wound site.

Where physiotherapy can work with body to prevent/improve maladaptive healing

The healing process occurs to form a functional scar to repair the injured tissue, and the aim of physiotherapy is to limit tissue damage and size of scar, produce quality scar tissue and maximise the efficiency of the healing process. The physiotherapeutic intervention used and the timing of the intervention are crucial. The consideration and appreciation of the healing process forms the basis of a rehabilitation programme, although an appreciation that many of our clients have come to us because the normal healing process has not occurred. It should also be noted that application of therapy at an inappropriate time can delay healing or produce non-functional scar tissue.

In the acute inflammatory stage, the focus of physiotherapy should be to restrict the inflammation, but not stop it. After the acute inflammatory stage (once the peak inflammatory response is reached), the focus should be to aid the reabsorption of the oedema.

After injury, the RICE (rest, ice, compression and elevation) principle is recommended for the first 2–3 days to control the cardinal signs of inflammation and aid resolution of the inflammatory stage.

Rest is encouraged to avoid putting physical stress through the early scar formation and new blood vessels, as these structures are fragile and disruption will prolong haemorrhage and the inflammatory process.

Ice is encouraged to reduce oedema, but the mechanism through which this occurs is unclear. Cold is thought to cause vasoconstriction, however research does not support this. Therefore, ice is believed to reduce cellular metabolic activity. The reduction in activity will reduce the oxygen requirements of the cells and reduce the release of inflammatory chemical mediators. Ice will also reduce the sensitivity of the nociceptors and therefore reduce pain.

Compression and elevation are used to control the amount of oedema. This is important to regain function as excess inflammatory exudate will increase the amount of fibrin in the area and increase the amount of scar tissue formed. This can be started immediately and continued for up to a week following injury in acute injuries. Compression can be applied by machines, bandaging or taping and massage (Figure 3.14).

There is an argument to include movement in the RICE principle as controlled mobilisation can stimulate the healing process. After the initial 24–48 hours following trauma, controlled pain-free movement should be encouraged and therapists can advise owners on the introduction of movement and the progression of movements to avoid overstressing the healing breach. In the early stages, this is likely to include gentle range of movement exercises to aid lymphatic drainage and reduce pain by stimulating mechanoreceptors. If mobilisation is not possible, then static contractions of muscles around the injury site help to reduce oedema and this can be done using neuromuscular electrical stimulation (NMES). The early use of electrical stimulation

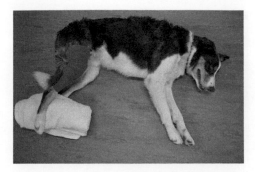

Figure 3.14 *Compression application.* Following acute injury, the application of compression will limit the amount of soft tissue swelling. By using a towel to support the distal leg, you can also elevate the leg quite easily.

can also help to reduce the amount of atrophy in muscular tissue around the wound site that has been immobilised through inhibition or spasm. Electrotherapy modalities are discussed in greater detail in Chapter 5.

Electrotherapy, such as pulsed electromagnetic field therapy (PEMFT) and transcutaneous electrical nerve stimulation (TENS), can be used in the first week for pain relief. Early use of electrical stimulation may also reduce the permeability of blood vessels and enhance protein synthesis, thus aiding the resolution of oedema and formation of fibrin clot.

The use of ultrasound (at a non-thermal setting) during angiogenesis can help rebuild the blood vessels; however, if set to produce a thermal effect, it can cause increased bleeding from the fragile vessels, and hence care is needed. Once the wound site has an established vascular system, the application of heat will aid the healing process by increasing cellular metabolic activity and circulation. These, in turn, will increase the exchange of nutrients and waste material. Heat is also useful in reducing any ongoing muscle spasm allowing the area to be gently moved.

Gentle stretching within the proliferation stage will prevent overcontraction of the wound by the action of myofibroblasts and prevent overadhesion between the wound edges. However, the stretching must be monitored carefully as the tensile strength is increasing in the stage and must not be pushed past its capacity. The synthesis of collagen reaches its peak between days 14 and 21 (depending on tissue type) and before this, the tension applied to the wound site must be pain-free. After this time, the tension applied can start to cause some discomfort, which will be indicated by the animal as slight resistance to movement. It is important to be very careful when assessing discomfort in the animal as some will be more stoical than others. If in any doubt it is always better to be more gentle as too vigorous too early will disrupt the healing breach. Gradually increasing the tension on a wound area will promote collagen synthesis. The more collagen within the breach by day 21, the quicker the return to function. Transverse friction massage (discussed in greater detail in Chapter 6) can help prevent excessive cross links within the collagen fibres. As the scar matures, the strength and depth of massage can be increased and more vigorous mobilisation is encouraged to stretch and maintain the mobility of the scar. Prolonged pressure from massage and friction massage can restore the balance of collagen synthesis and

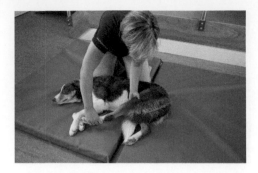

Figure 3.15 *Passive range of movement.* The stretching of the healing lesion in the proliferation stage will promote the alignment of collagen fibres and improve the tensile strength of the scar tissue being formed.

reabsorption. Therefore, where excessive scar tissue has formed, this can be useful in mobilising adhesions and facilitating the reabsorption of the collagen.

During the proliferation phase, an increase in range of movement (ROM) should be encouraged through passive stretching and active ROM. This will promote the orientation of fibres and it should be progressed through an exercise programme (or rehabilitation programme, see Chapter 8 for more details) to achieve full pain-free ROM (Figure 3.15).

Electrotherapy, such as laser, ultrasound and PEMFT will aid the synthesis of collagen and promote contraction of the wound through increasing the activity of myofibroblasts (further details in Chapter 7).

In the remodelling phase, if excessive adhesions have occurred, dynamic and passive stretching of these is extremely important. Ultrasound can also be included to stretch the connective tissue to aid the reduction of these adhesions and promote an increase in range of movement.

The treatment aims of the remodelling stage are the same as the proliferation stage, but we can apply greater pressure to the healing breach and increase the resistance applied to muscular tissues to increase the strength of these. In a chronic injury, where a mature scar has been formed but is causing dysfunction, all the techniques used will cause a mild to moderate amount of discomfort as maladaptive healing will have occurred and the aim is to restore normal movement.

CHAPTER 4

Clinical examination

Clinical examination should identify problems, both primary and secondary, that a patient may have, so that a suitable treatment plan can be drawn up. It is divided into history and ancillary information (Subjective), a thorough physical examination (Objective), Analysis of the findings and drawing up of a Plan (SOAP). Included in the plan should be outcome measures to monitor the success of the treatment protocol. The treatment plan and outcome measures will change as the animal progresses through recovery. Reassessments at regular intervals are required.

A thorough clinical examination is essential and should not be rushed. A typical examination with history taking, hands-on examination, analysis of finding and the drawing up of a plan will usually take 1–1.5 hours.

Subjective

History
Any clinical examination should always start with a thorough history taking. Many indicators and snippets of useful information can be gleaned from a good questioning about the history.

Baseline information
Baseline information, such as age, breed, sex and neutered state, can give vital clues. For example, an 8-month-old Labrador with front leg lameness should throw up some possibilities that should be considered at the physical examination.

How long has the problem been going on? Is the problem recent, chronic or recurring?

Which leg does the owner/referring veterinarian think the dog is lame on?

Does the dog ever carry the leg? Which leg?

Is the lameness a recurring problem? If so, when did the problem first appear? Have there been any previous injuries to the area? How has the problem responded to treatment? Have they sought any other treatment and what type of treatment (chiropractic/physiotherapy/hydrotherapy)? How did the problem respond to this treatment?

Is the patient on any medication? What response did the patient have to the medication? This is particularly important with NSAIDS. Poor response to NSAIDS

Practical Physiotherapy for Small Animal Practice, First Edition.
Edited by David Prydie and Isobel Hewitt.
© 2015 John Wiley & Sons, Ltd. Published 2015 by John Wiley & Sons, Ltd.
Companion Website: www.wiley.com/go/practical-physiotherapy-for-small-animals

is common in certain conditions. It is also important when drawing up a treatment plan. In many chronic conditions, the inflammatory response has subsided before healing is complete. Part of treatment, for example, shockwave, may be to restart the inflammatory process to encourage blood supply. NSAIDS will counteract this restarted inflammation, and hence it may be better to provide pain relief with drugs other than NSAIDS (see Chapter 10).

Exercise

What distance does the dog walk on a daily basis? Is this one long walk or is it broken into a series of smaller walks? Is the dog on a lead or free running? Does the owner encourage ball games? What is the terrain? Are there other dogs in the household or on the walks? What age are these dogs? When were they acquired? Does the time fit in with when the lameness started? Does the problem improve or deteriorate with exercise? Is the patient stiff on rising after a rest following exercise? Does the patient warm out of the limp? How willing is the patient to exercise?

Diet and supplements

Is the plain of nutrition appropriate for the animal's stage in life? Is the nutrition sufficient to support recovery? Is the animal being overfed or receiving lots of extra titbits or treats? Is the patient receiving sufficient dose supplements that may enhance recovery? For example, Omega 3/EPA.

Does the animal have any other medical conditions, for example, endocrine (hypothyroidism, Cushing's disease) that may affect the musculoskeletal system, or other issues such as heart disease that may affect the choice of modalities? (see Chapter 5)

Environment

Is the animal a family pet or does it compete at any sports? For example, agility, fly ball, obedience or used as a gun dog (Figure 4.1). In this situation, it may be useful to have the owner video the dog at work and review this at the clinical examination. Remember the canine athlete sustains injuries not normally seen in the pet animal.

Have the owners owned the animal from a pup/kitten or is the pet a rescue? Were there any problems during the growing phase?

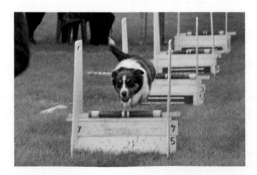

Figure 4.1   The canine athlete, in this case, a fly ball dog, sustains injuries not normally seen in pet dogs.

Establish what type of motor vehicle the owners have and where the dog travels in the vehicle. Jumping down from a 4×4 could have significant impact on front leg lameness both as cause and during recovery.

What type of flooring do the owners have? Does the dog have to walk across slippery or laminate floors? This could be significant with repeated falls and would need to be addressed as part of the treatment plan.

Demeanour

Is the patient dull or depressed? Does the animal seek attention or is it withdrawn and avoids contact with people and other animals? Has there been any change in the animal's mood or behaviour?

Ancillary information

Try to find the X-ray report, any blood tests as well as the surgical report including any problems at surgery. All of these will give valuable information that can be used to draw up a treatment plan.

Objective

Observe the dog in standing. Assess if the joints are correctly aligned. Is the carpus or hock dropped? Is the leg outwardly or inwardly rotated?
Note: Slight outward rotation of the front leg in standing is normal (Figure 4.2).

Weight and body condition score should be recorded. These should be recorded at each subsequent visit. Is the patient under- or overweight? Is this contributing to the problem?

Make the dog sit. Observe the sit. Is one back leg rotated outwards? (Figure 4.3) Make the dog come to a stand. Observe the position of the legs. Normally, the dog should stand square with a leg in each corner. Is one leg out of position? Sometimes the affected leg is held out of position. This is called triangulation (Figure 4.4).

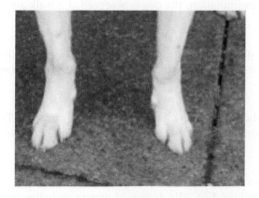

Figure 4.2   Slight outward rotation of the feet at a stand is normal.

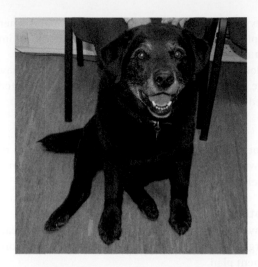

Figure 4.3   Observe the dog at a sit and note any asymmetry.

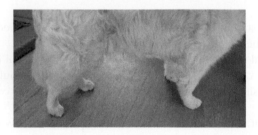

Figure 4.4   Often the three sound legs form a right-angled triangle while the affected leg is out of alignment.

Gait analysis

For this part of the examination, the dog is observed at a walk and at a trot.

Gait

Only the basic gait observation of a walk, trot and pace will be discussed here. For more information on other gaits and gait analysis, please see further reading.

Walk

At the walk, there should be 3 feet on the ground at any one time. The normal footfall is LH, LF, RH and RF (Figure 4.5). The centre of gravity stays central.

Pace

With a pace, the two legs on the same side will move forward together. Footfall is LF + LH, RF + RH (Figure 4.6). The centre of gravity switches from left to right as the dog moves forward. This is an incorrect and inefficient gait. A large number of dogs will pace. These dogs often have issues in the paraspinal muscles. Dogs that pace

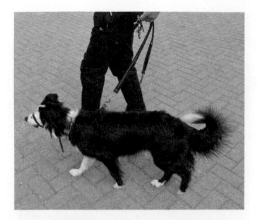

Figure 4.5 *The walk.* Three feet are on the ground at any one time. To start walking, a dog first lifts its left back leg and moves it under its body.

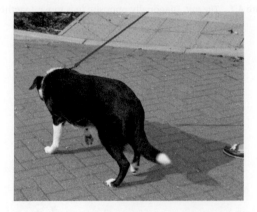

Figure 4.6 *Pacing.* Both left feet are off the ground at the same time. This is an inefficient gait as the centre of gravity is constantly shifting from side to side.

may be doing so because of lameness, but many will never have learnt how to walk properly. For correction of pacing, see Chapter 8.

Tip: If you are having trouble deciding if a dog is pacing by looking from the side, watch the dog walking away from you. If you can see the pads of the two right or two left feet at the same time, the dog is pacing.

Trot

In the trot, the two diagonal legs move forward together. The footfall is LF + RH, RF + LH (Figure 4.7). The back foot on each side should land almost in the same place as the front foot on that side. At the trot, the placing of the foot moves more central, creating a 'V' shape with the legs (Figure 4.8).

Crabbing

Crabbing is where the back foot passes beyond the front foot on the same side, passing either medially or laterally to the front foot. Crabbing may occur at the walk or at

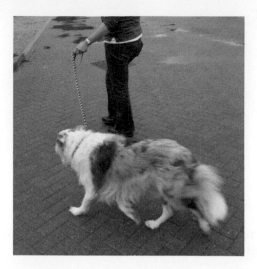

Figure 4.7 *The trot.* Diagonally opposite legs move together.

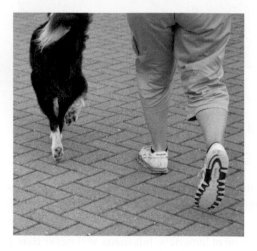

Figure 4.8 At the trot, the two back legs and two front legs move more medially, creating a V shape.

the trot. Some dogs will have no option but to crab. For example, the GSD with the long sloping back and angulated rear legs. In this situation, the rear leg stride is longer than that of the front leg. Other dogs will crab as a result of lameness or musculoskeletal problems. For example, a dog with a painful right hip may crab to the right, as the right back leg will have less distance to travel than if walking straight. The iliopsoas muscle can be used to advance the leg with little flexion and extension of the right hip.

The dog should be observed walking away and coming towards and from both sides in both walk and trot.

The dog should then be made to circle clockwise and anticlockwise at both walk and trot.

For front leg issues, look any nodding of the head. The head normally nods when the sound front leg hits the ground.

For rear leg issues, look for any lifting of the affected leg. Observe if there is a swaggering gait. (For example, a Labrador puppy with HD that has a 'sexy' wiggle or a Marilyn Monroe walk according to the owners. The puppy is actually in pain.)

Note the tail carriage. Does it hang freely and stay central or is it arched or move to one side?

Tip: Watch the tail. If the spinal muscles are being used to advance the pelvic leg, the tail will swing to that side.

Note the head carriage. Is the head held in the normal position or is it dropped?

Try to observe each leg in turn to see if each joint is being flexed and extended. Is there any weight shifting either from one side to the other or from back to front or vice versa?

Is the gait uncoordinated? Is there crossing of legs? Is this a neurological problem?

Listen for any scuffing of nails and try to identify which foot or feet are involved.

Tip: Get an iPhone or Android movie application that allows instant review in slow motion. We use SloPro.

Range of motion

Range of motion of a joint is defined as the degree of motion that occurs when the bones comprising a joint move about the joint axis. Range of motion may be passive or active.

With passive range of motion (PROM), the patient plays no role in the movement. Movement of the joint about its axis is initiated and carried out completely by the operator. There is no muscle contraction on the part of the dog.

Active range of motion (AROM) is initiated and carried out by the patient. It requires muscle contraction. PROM can be measured using a goniometer and specific bony landmarks. A goniometer is a protractor with a fixed arm, a fulcrum and a moving arm (Figure 4.9). Different sizes of goniometer are required for different breeds

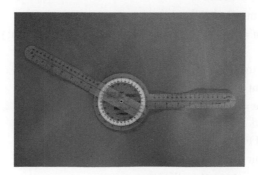

Figure 4.9   A goniometer consists of a 360° protractor with a central fulcrum, a fixed arm and a movable arm.

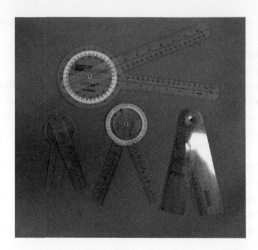

Figure 4.10   Examples of different types and sizes of goniometer.

and joints (Figure 4.10). The fix arm is placed on the proximal bony landmark. The fulcrum is placed over the joint axis. The moving arm is placed on the distal bony landmark. The operator then moves the joint through flexion and extension noting the degrees of motion on the goniometer

The bony landmarks for measuring PROM in the dog are shown below.

Shoulder flexion and extension (Figure 4.11(a)).

Fulcrum = acromion process.

Fixed proximal arm = scapula spine.

Distal moving point = lateral epicondyle.

Elbow (Figure 4.11(b)).

Fulcrum = lateral epicondyle.

Fixed proximal point = greater tubercle.

Moving distal point = ulna styloid.

Carpus (Figure 4.11(c)).

Fulcrum = ulna carpal bone.

Fixed proximal point = radial head.

Distal moving point = lateral aspect of fifth metacarpo-phalangeal joint.

Hip (Figure 4.11(d)).

Fulcrum = greater trochanter.

Proximal fixed point = wing of ilium.

Distal moving point = lateral femoral epicondyle.

Stifle (Figure 4.11.(e)).

Fulcrum = Head of Fibula.

Proximal fixed point = greater trochanter.

Distal moving Point = Lateral malleolus.

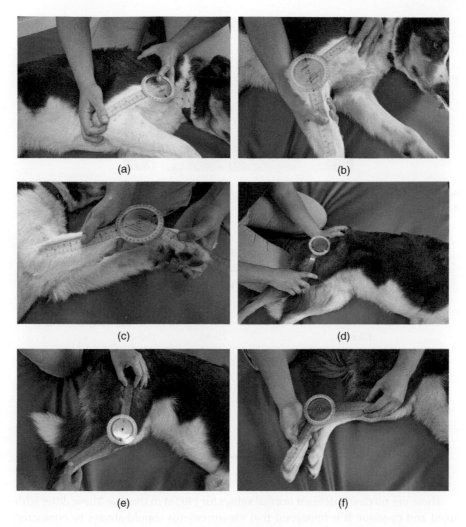

Figure 4.11   (a) Measurement of shoulder ROM. (b) Measurement of elbow ROM. (c) Measurement of carpus ROM. (d) Measurement of hip ROM. (e) Measurement of stifle ROM. (f) Measurement of hock ROM.

Hock (Figure 4.11.(f)).

Fulcrum = Lateral Malleolus.

Fixed proximal point = Head of Fibula.

Distal moving point = Lateral aspect of fifth metatarso-phalangeal joint.

Shoulder abduction (Figure 4.12).

Fulcrum = glenoid tubercle of scapula.

Fixed proximal arm = cranial border of scapula.

Distal moving point = cranial aspect of humerus.

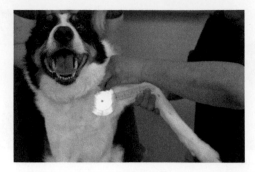

Figure 4.12   Measurement of shoulder abduction angle. This should always be compared with the other side.

Table 4.1   'Normal' PROM values in the dog.

Joint	Flexion (°)	Extension (°)
Shoulder	50–65	150–160
Elbow	25–40	150–165
Carpus	30–40	0–15
Hip	50–70	165
Stifle	25–40	145–160
Hock	30–40	160–170
Shoulder abduction 20–45°		

There are no clearly defined normal values for PROM in the dog. These differ with breed and operator. It is important that measurements should always be compared with the contralateral leg and any abnormalities recorded (Table 4.1).

Flexibility

When measuring or assessing PROM, it is important to take into account the flexibility of the muscles that flex and extend the joint. Flexibility refers to the length of a muscle. Reduced flexibility is the result of tight or shortened muscles. This is a pathological condition with various causes.

Flexibility is a function of muscle, and range of motion is a function of a joint. There is no such thing as a flexible joint. Reduced flexibility often occurs in muscles that cross two joints. This is particularly important and well demonstrated in the shoulder and elbow.

When measuring PROM of a shoulder or an elbow, it is important to note the position of the other joint (flexion, extension or neutral). The PROM reading obtained for shoulder extension will be considerably different if the elbow is flexed rather than extended. This is due to the flexibility of the long head of triceps.

The biceps brachii muscle originates from the supraglenoid tubercle of the scapula. The tendon of origin runs through the bicipital groove between the lesser and greater tubercles of the humerus. It is held in place by a transverse ligament. The *single* bellied muscle then runs down the cranial aspect of the humerus before bifurcating to insert on medial coronoid process of ulna and the radial head. It therefore crosses both shoulder and elbow joints. Its actions are to flex the elbow and extend the shoulder. Innervation is by the musculocutaneous nerve (Chapter 2).

The other two joint muscle in the shoulder and elbow is the long head of triceps brachii. The triceps brachii muscle consists of *four* muscle bellies in the dog. The medial, lateral and accessory heads all originate from proximal humerus and insert onto the olecranon process of the ulna. Their action is to extend the elbow. The *long* head of triceps brachii, which forms most of the muscle mass of the caudal aspect of the humerus and is the main antigravity muscle in the fore leg, originates from caudal border of scapula and inserts with the other three heads onto the olecranon. Its action is also to extend the elbow and *also to flex the shoulder* (Chapter 2).

End feels

An end feel is a sensation the operator experiences when a joint reaches the end of its available range of motion.

Normal end feels

- Bony or Hard – elbow extension. Motion is prevented by bony obstruction.
- Soft Tissue – elbow flexion. Further movement is prohibited by muscle mass.
- Capsular or Firm – normal carpal extension. There is a firm feeling but with a springy elasticity or give.

Abnormal end feels

- Bony (e.g. hip) with OA with osteophytes.
- Springy block – rebound effect before the expected end of range. Often indicates problem within the joint (e.g. meniscal injury in the stifle).
- Muscle spasm – sudden hard end feel due to muscle spasm often accompanied by pain (e.g. biceps brachii contracture).
- Capsular – further motion is restricted tight or fibrosed joint capsule (e.g. OA joint).
- Empty – no end point or resistance, patient stops motion because of pain.

Summary of things that affect the ROM of a joint

- Pain
- Joint capsule fibrosis
- Fascial tissue
- Musculo-tendinous tissue
  - Adaptive shortening
  - Trigger points
- Bone – osteophytes
- Swelling

- ○ Intra-articular – effusion
- ○ Extra-articular – oedema
- Meniscus
- Surgery

Muscle mass

Muscle mass can be measured using a girthometer or Gulick. A Gulick consists of a tape measure with a spring-loaded tension device on one end. The operator measures the circumference of the leg at a set place and tensions the tape using the spring-loaded device. When one red ball shows in viewing chamber, there is 2 oz. (50 g) of pressure. When two red balls show, there is 4 oz. (100 g) of pressure (Figure 4.13).

When measuring muscle mass, try to use a repeatable place. Common sites would be thigh girth at its widest point. In the immediate post-operative case that is shaved, a reference line can be drawn on the skin to ensure measurement at the same site. Always compare with the contralateral side. Although somewhat basic, this technique does give a good objective outcome measure. It is extremely popular with clients to monitor recovery in their animal.

Hands-on examination

Even if the lameness is obvious, it is important to carry out a full examination of the whole of the musculoskeletal system. If a dog comes in on, three legs do not jump to the non-weight-bearing leg. There will be secondary problems associated with compensating for walking on three legs. These problems must be identified and addressed.

Before laying hands on the patient, try to make friends by offering treats or toys. Try to get the patient and the owner to relax. Light hands are the order of the day here. Abnormalities that you are trying to detect may be quite subtle, such as changes in the tone of paraspinal muscles. A heavy-handed technique will miss vital information.

Tip: DAP/Feliway diffusers in the consult room may help calm patients.

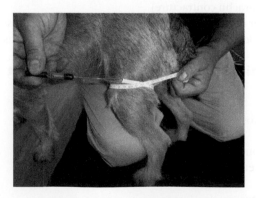

Figure 4.13   Girthometer or Gulick being used to measure muscle mass.

Tip: During the examination, we are looking for subtle clues that may indicate pain or discomfort. Often if a painful area is palpated, the dog will lick its lips or look away from the examiner. Other signs may be a change in respiration rate, either speeding up or more often, stopping panting. Remember for a dog to show pain in the wild pack situation is a sign of weakness, and hence dogs will try to conceal injury or pain (see Chapter 10).

Work out your own examination technique and follow for each and every dog. Some examiners like to have the patient in lateral recumbency and work down one side before rolling the patient over and working down the other side. Others prefer to examine the dog in standing as it is easier to compare contra-lateral side.

Personal technique (DP). Starting at temporo-mandibular joint (TMJ) on both sides, assess for signs of abnormal movement, clicking or pain. Move the hands to palpate the wings of the atlas, the axis and dorsal cervical area. Move laterally to identify the transverse processes of C3–5. Any pain or trigger points are noted. Go down to thoracic inlet and palpate the large transverse processes of C6. Moving caudally and slightly medially, displace the trachea to feel C6/7 discs space. Gently apply pressure and watch for any reaction. Palpate the first few ribs in their entirety. Problems in this area are underdiagnosed and are not uncommon, particularly in obedience dogs on the left-hand side.

Palpate between the scapulae and gradually work down the paraspinal muscles. Note any twitching and any change in muscle tone. Continue down to dorsal wings of ilium. The L7 vertebra lies direct between the wings of ilium. From L7, move back up the lumbar spine feeling the spinous and transverse processes up to the thoracic spine. Feel for the anticlinal vertebra. Moving back to the L7, feel for the small dorsal spine of L7 and drop off the back of the vertebra to palpate L/S junction. Apply gentle pressure in the midline and to the facet area on both sides. Palpate the sacrum and coccygeal vertebrae. Holding one side of the ilium by its ventral and dorsal borders in one hand, gently move the ilium after stabilising the sacrum with the other hand. Note any pain or reaction. Try to estimate the degree of movement. Repeat on the other side. This is to check for sacroiliac issues that are a common finding. Gently palpate the piriformis muscles that run from sacrum/Co1 to greater trochanter. Gently pull on the tail and shift it to the right and left noting any resistance or discomfort.

Gently run the hands over the rib cage and abdomen noting muscle tone and any trigger points.

Front leg

Gently lift one front leg and then replace. Lift the other front leg. Are they the same? Is there any weight shifting? Is one leg taking more weight than the other? Observe the way the dog is standing on the leg. Are the joints all aligned or is weight being shifted medially or laterally?

Do a basic conscious proprioception reflex in all cases. If these are slow or absent, do a full neurological examination after the hands-on examination. Neurological examination is covered in Chapter 7.

Foot

Observe the feet and digits. Is the foot flat? This may be 'normal' in an old dog, but may be significant in a younger animal (Figure 4.14). Are the digits curled under? If

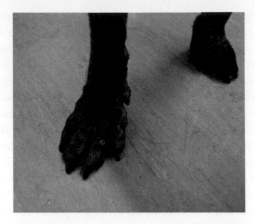

Figure 4.14   Flat feet in older dogs are common.

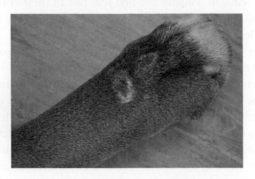

Figure 4.15   Lick granulomas often indicate an underlying problem.

so, how easy are they to straighten? Is there contracture of the flexor tendons? Look for any signs of licking or any lick granulomata (Figure 4.15).

Position the dog in a stand. Start with digits and flex and extend each in turn. Check the nails for any nail bed infection, wear or bleeding. A lot of dogs will have 'tickly' feet and may resent examination. This must be distinguished from reaction to an area of pain. Are the other feet sensitive? Pull gently on each digit. Palpate the phalangeal joints and note any exostoses. Record any redness or swelling and any discoloured fur. Look for any corns on the pads and any cuts or discharging sinuses.

Displace the main pad caudally and gently palpate the sesamoid bones of MC/P junction. Flex and extend P3/MC junction. Note the end feel and any restriction of movement or pain. Note the presence or absence of dewclaws.

Carpus

Record any medial or lateral deviation of the carpus. Flex and extend the carpus noting the end feel and range of motion. If there is a reduction or increase in the ROM, then this should be measured and the degrees of flexion and extension recorded. Try to establish what is restricting/increasing ROM. Is it soft tissue, bone or pain?

Palpate the radial and ulna styloids noting any abnormalities. With the carpus in flexion, palpate the radial and ulnar carpal bones followed by the numbered carpal bones. Try to assess the state of the joint capsule noting any effusion or thickening. Check the integrity of the co-lateral ligaments by abducting and adducting the foot while stabilising distal radius and ulna. Palpate the accessory carpal bone, its covering pad and its ligamentous attachments. If any abnormalities are detected, these are compared with the contralateral leg.

Elbow and shoulder

Flex and extend the elbow again noting ROM, end feel or crepitus. If ROM is reduced, measure it at this point. Rotate the radius and ulna medially and laterally in flexion, in a neutral position and in extension, paying particular attention to loading of the coronoid process of ulna. Palpate the flexors and extensors muscles for any trigger points or areas of altered tone or tenderness. Feel the olecranon and insertion of the triceps mm. Fully flex the elbow and press on the anconeal area. During elbow examination, try to keep the shoulder in a neutral position. Remember the biceps brachii and long head of triceps have actions on both joints.

With the elbow in flexion, palpate the triceps mm. This is a common site for trigger points or areas of tightness. With the elbow still held in flexion, extend the shoulder thereby stretching the long head of triceps. Feel for any tight bands of tissue around the triceps, particularly on the medial side.

Now perform a biceps stress test by flexing the shoulder and extending the elbow (Figure 4.16). In this position, apply gentle pressure to the tendon of origin of the biceps brachii. Dogs with pain in the biceps will often lick their lips and look away. Note how far the elbow extends and compare this to what would be expected in the normal dog. Note the end feel. Reduce some of the extension on the elbow and then palpate the belly of biceps for tone, trigger points and pain.

Tip: A positive biceps stress test does not necessarily mean a shoulder issue. Remember biceps brachii inserts onto radial head and coronoid process of ulna. Dogs with elbow dysplasia will often have a positive biceps test.

Identify deltoid tuberosity on the humerus and palpate the deltoid muscles. Work medially to 180° opposite the deltoid tuberosity and gently palpate for tendon of

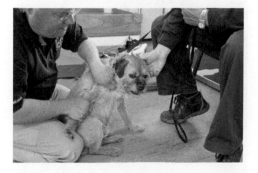

Figure 4.16 *Biceps stress test.* Flex the shoulder, extend the elbow and apply gentle pressure to the biceps tendon. Watch for any licking or changes in breathing pattern.

insertion of latissimus dorsi and teres major. This is high up in the dog's axilla. Great care is needed when examining this area, as it is very sensitive. Usually, this tendon is difficult to palpate but if there are problems, the tendon is much more obvious and tight. Palpation will usually cause rippling over the trunk as the latissimus dorsi muscle is irritated.

Identify dorsal border of scapula and work down the spinous process identifying supraspinatus and noting any muscle atrophy. Palpate caudal to the spine and assess muscle mass. Identify acromion process and try to gently palpate the tendon of insertion of infraspinatus. Now go to the cranial aspect of the shoulder joint, palpate the insertion of supraspinatus and apply slight pressure noting any reaction. Palpate the biceps tendon and bicipital groove. Palpate the pectoral girdle noting tone. Often in shoulder problems, the pectorals are clamped down restricting shoulder movement.

Flex and extend the shoulder with the elbow in a neutral position recording any abnormality and measure if required. Try to abduct the shoulder by keeping scapula stationary with one hand and gently taking the elbow away from the body. Any increase in abduction angle is measured and recorded. The end feel is also noted. It is very important to identify the end feel in this situation as the normal abduction angle varies greatly in the dog. If abnormality is suspected, then it should be compared with the contralateral leg.

See how the dog reacts to inward rotation of the shoulder throughout range of motion. This is repeated for outward rotation.

I would now measure muscle mass of the shoulder girdle and compare with the other side (Figure 4.17).

Back leg

Again, starting with the foot, repeat the examination as per the front foot. Working up the leg, palpate the flexor tendons noting any pain or swelling. Look at the position of the toes. Are they curled under? Is there any contracture of the flexor tendons?

Hock/Tarsus

Palpate the tarso-metatarsal joint and check for any abnormal movement. Check the integrity of the intertarsal ligaments. Palpate the medial and lateral malleoli and

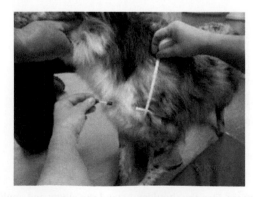

Figure 4.17 Measuring shoulder muscle mass with a Gulick.

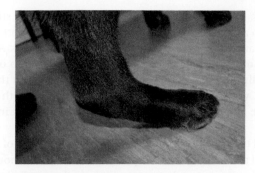

Figure 4.18   Look for dropping of the hock and palpate the Achilles tendon for any thickening.

calcaneus. Check range of motion of the tarsocrural joint, measuring any reduction or increase. End feel is again important here. Any bony proliferations should also be recorded. Now palpate the Achilles tendon, feeling for any thickening (Figure 4.18). Palpate the insertion of the deep part of the tendon onto calcaneus. Palpate up the tendon to the gastrocnemius muscle bellies. Try to identify the superficial digital flexor tendon running in a small groove on the tip of calcaneus. Flex and extend the hock while holding the stifle fixed in a neutral position, palpating the gastrocnemius muscles right up to their origin. Also palpate the cranial tibial muscle. Any pain or tightness should be recorded.

Stifle
Palpate the stifle joint feeling for any thickening or joint effusion. Check the medial side of proximal tibia for any buttress formation. Holding the stifle in a neutral position, flex the hock causing tension in the gastrocnemius muscles. Feel for any movement in the stifle while doing this. Place the thumb of one hand on the tibia, just caudal to the head of fibula and place the index finger on the tibial tuberosity. With the other three fingers, grasp the tibia. Place the thumb of the other hand on lateral fabella and the index finger on patella. The remaining fingers grasp the femur. Now attempt to pull the femur cranially and then caudally (Figure 4.19). Any excess

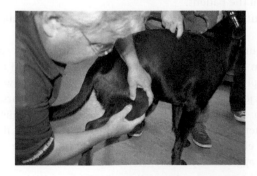

Figure 4.19   Forward drawer test for checking the integrity of the cruciate ligaments.

movement is noted. Carry out this forward drawer test with the stifle in extension, in a neutral position and in flexion. In doing so, the integrity of both the caudolateral and craniomedial bands of the cranial cruciate ligament is tested. At this stage, also check the integrity of the co-lateral ligaments by gently trying to open up the joint medially and laterally. Any excess movement is noted along with the end feels.

I (DP) use the Cyriax D stroke to test meniscal integrity. With stifle in flexion, attempt to write the letter D with lower leg. Any pain or clicking indicates a meniscal injury.

Flex and extend the stifle several times and note the tracking of the patella. Note range of motion and measure if there is any reduction. End feels should also be noted. Put the stifle in full extension and attempt to luxate the patella both medially and laterally. Any movement, grating or discomfort is recorded. Try to assess the grade of luxation if present.

The head of fibula is palpated along with the tendon of origin of the long digital extensor.

Run the hands over the quadriceps mass while flexing and extending the stifle. Note any restriction of movement, trigger points or signs of atrophy. Now palpate the hamstring group, feeling the bellies and tendons of semimembranosus and semitendinosus. Palpate the belly of gracilis muscle noting any swelling or thickening. Follow the belly down to palpate the tendon of insertion on the tibia, feeling for any thickening. Extend the stifle and hock. Gently push the foot towards the head, creating a stretch on the hamstrings. Resistance and discomfort are noted.

Measure muscle mass at the maximum thigh girth and compare with the contralateral side.

Hip

Start by flexing hip and noting any resistance. Then slowly bring the hip into a neutral position and then finally into extension. Any reduction in ROM is noted and measured. End feel is also recorded, as is any discomfort or pain. With the hip in extension, gently inwardly rotate the stifle. This will stretch iliopsoas muscle. Any reduced ROM, resistance or discomfort is noted. The hip is now externally rotated in flexion and extension.

Gluteals are palpated for any abnormalities and an assessment of any atrophy is made by comparing with the other side and what might be considered the norm for the breed and age of the patient.

Pectineus is identified in the medial thigh. The hip is gently abducted while palpating pectineus.

The wings of ilium are identified along with the short dorsal spinous process of L7 that sits between them. Identify the L/S space by dropping off the caudal border of L7. Now gently press on the L/S space and note reaction. Move slightly laterally to palpate the facet joints. Now place the right arm under metatarsal areas and flex, hock, stifle and hip. With the legs in this compressed state, stabilise the body of L7 with the left and then gently rock with the right arm. This action flexes and extends L/S junction while eliminating hip, stifle or hock movement. Be careful, dogs with L/S pain may react aggressively to this test.

Analysis

A list of problems should now be drawn up. These should include findings from the subjective history, ancillary tests and lifestyle information, as well as the gait observations, objective markers and hands-on examination.

Plan

From the analysis of the list of problems, a treatment plan is drawn up that will last until the next assessment. The examination will then be repeated, a new set of problems identified and a new plan devised. The plan should include goals of treatment that are agreed with the owner. We use SMART (*S*pecific *M*easurable *A*chievable *R*elevant *T*imeframe) goals. These give a clear outline of how treatment will progress in a certain time frame, allow realistic goals to be set which is especially useful if the patient may not be able to return to full athletic ability, provide motivation for the owner to comply with rehabilitation program and highlight any problems quickly.

Outcome measures

These may be subjective or objective and are designed to quantify and monitor recovery. Any deviation from the set outcome measure or changes to expected progression of treatment should be investigated.

Examples of subjective outcome measures would be changes to the dog's demeanour, or how bright the owner feels the dog is. Other subjective measures may involve things that the dog used to be able to do but has not done for a while. These may include going upstairs, getting on the furniture, getting into the car or playing with toys or other dogs.

Objective outcome measures may include changes in the range of motion of a joint as measured with a goniometer, changes in muscle girth as measured with a Gulick and changes in stamina as measured by the distance the dog is able to walk.

Outcome measures will change as the patient progresses through the treatment protocols. It is therefore important that re-examinations are carried out at regular intervals and that new outcome targets are set.

Following is a typical SOAP for a dog that has had a left cruciate operated on 2 days before the initial physiotherapy examination.

Subjective

A 6-year-old MN Chocolate Labrador Retriever 39 kg (86 lb) pet dog. One other dog (FN 4 years old Yellow Labrador Retriever) and two young children (6 and 8 years old) in the house. Dog went 10/10 lame 2 days before having surgery, but owner reports stiffness on rising on LH for the previous 6 weeks. The dog is fed on a supermarket own label complete dog food. Normally exercised for 20 minutes twice daily, longer at weekends. Vehicle is a 4 × 4. Dog travels in the back with the other dog and jumps down when the back is opened. The dog lives in a single-storey building. There are laminate and vinyl floors in the kitchen and hall.

LH CCL repaired by TPLO technique 2 days ago. No complications at surgery reported. Osteophytes and joint effusion noted on X-ray. Osteophytes noted at surgery. On NSAIDS and fentanyl patch.

Objective

Body condition score 7/9. Dog BAR. Pain control adequate. Toe touching LH at a stand. Lame at walk 10/10. Using iliopsoas to advance LH. Wound with mild degree of post-operative swelling left stifle. Reduced ROM left stifle only 45 degrees of motion. End feel empty due to pain. Large medial buttress obvious on left proximal tibia, smaller medial buttress palpable on right tibia. Muscle thigh girth RH 50 cm, LH 41 cm. Weight shifted to the right and forwards. Increase in tone and irritability (trigger points) in paraspinal muscles T6 – L7 both sides. Discomfort on iliopsoas stretch LH. Positive biceps stress test RF. Pectoral muscles increased tone more so on the right.

Analysis

Dog is overweight. Flooring and lifestyle could compromise recovery. LH CCL repair with TPLO. Muscle wasting LH greater than would be expected from only 4 days of 10/10 lame. Stiffness on rising for 6 weeks and findings on X-ray and at surgery suggests established joint pathology. Right stifle is showing early signs of cruciate disease. The dog is using its iliopsoas and paraspinal muscles to advance the LH. Weight is shifted forward, which is causing problems with the right biceps brachii muscle and pectoral girdle.

Plan

Continue pain medication and monitor pain scores.

Diet
Weight loss. Target weight 34 kg (75 lb.) Advise weight-reducing diet or cutting ration by one-third and replacing with cooked pumpkin or butternut squash. Suggest changing diet to a better protein source than the current food. Advise the addition of Omega 3/EPA to support joint health but it must be remembered that this is a fat and weight loss is the priority initially.

Environment
Advise rugs and runners for the slippery flooring and a ramp for the car.

Exercise

Advise 5 minutes toilet breaks on the lead three times daily. No playing with other dogs or children.

Physiotherapy

Advise icing of the wound for 15 minutes three times daily for the next 48 hours. Attempt PROM of the stifle but only within comfort range. Three repetitions twice daily. Advise flexion and extension of digits and hock holding each position for 10 seconds. Three repetitions twice daily

Laser (see Chapter 5) wound, joint and osteotomy site, right biceps brachii muscle and tendon, pectorals, iliopsoas and paraspinal muscles, daily for 3 days. The laser treatment is then dropped to every other day for the next 7 days.

EMS (see Chapter 5) to quadriceps and hamstring muscle: groups. Machine set on synchronous for 10 minutes every other day.

Outcome measures

By 14 days post op., reduction in joint swelling; increase ROM in left stifle by 15° with no pain; reduction of trigger points in paraspinals and pectorals. Dog able to bear weight on LH for 30 seconds unassisted.

Follow-up

Reassess in 10 days. The re-examination would focus mainly on the findings of the first examination. A new plan would be drawn up and new outcome measures set. These would include weight-loss targets, increase in ROM and muscle girth.

CHAPTER 5

Modalities

Modalities are the physical entities used as part of a treatment plan. Many of these modalities introduce an energy source to the body to stimulate or support the healing process. These include thermotherapy and cryotherapy (the application or removal of heat), electrical muscle stimulation (electricity), laser therapy (light), ultrasound therapy (sound), pulsed electromagnetic field therapy (magnetism), extracorporeal shockwave therapy (pressure) and hydrotherapy (water).

Superficial hot and cold therapies

Superficial cold therapy (cryotherapy)
Indications
Cryotherapy is most often used in the acute phase of an injury or immediately post operatively. It can also be used in exercise-related injury.

Application of a cold pack to an area will reduce blood flow to that area. Cryotherapy has been shown to interfere with pain transmission. It also reduces oxygen demand from the surrounding tissues and will help reduce swelling. If cryotherapy is applied under pressure, this results in greater reduction in swelling and reduced pain scores.

Skin will show a 10°C drop in temperature after the application of an ice pack within 15 minutes. Subcutaneous tissue will take over 30 minutes to show a similar temperature drop and muscle will take much longer.

Cryotherapy can be applied in several forms such as crushed ice in a bag, bag of frozen peas and special cold packs that contain a gel that remains flexible when cold (Figure 5.1). The cold source should never be placed directly onto the animal and should always be wrapped in a damp towel or similar.

Tip: Ranges of wraps of different sizes and for different joints are available. The wraps have pockets for ice packs. These can be strapped around the area of injury without the need for someone to hold the pack in place (Figure 5.2).

Systems are also available that deliver cold therapy and pressure at the same time. The system consists of a series of different-sized wraps for various joints connected to a reservoir that holds ice-cold water. The wraps are secured around the relevant joint. Ice-cold water is then pumped into the wrap under pressure. After a few minutes, the water is exchanged for fresh ice-cold water from the reservoir. This system is particularly effective at controlling post-operative swelling.

Practical Physiotherapy for Small Animal Practice, First Edition.
Edited by David Prydie and Isobel Hewitt.
© 2015 John Wiley & Sons, Ltd. Published 2015 by John Wiley & Sons, Ltd.
Companion Website: www.wiley.com/go/practical-physiotherapy-for-small-animals

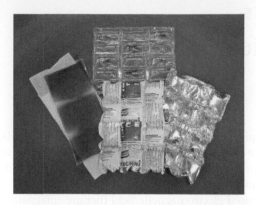

Figure 5.1   Keep a variety of ice packs in the freezer. Make sure the frozen product does not come into direct contact with the patient.

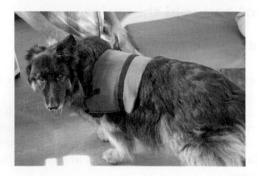

Figure 5.2   Wraps of different sizes with pockets for ice packs are available. (Canine Icer – see useful websites.)

Superficial hot therapy (thermotherapy)
Indications
Superficial heat is often used in chronic conditions such as OA and can also be useful for reducing muscle spasm. It promotes blood flow to an area, reduces pain and increases joint and soft-tissue flexibility. Superficial heat will penetrate about 1–2 cm in depth. Sources of heat include a damp towel placed in the microwave, wheat bags, heat mats, gel packs heated in hot water and special hot packs that generate heat on the mixing of two chemicals. Again a towel or similar should be placed between the hot pack and the animal's body.

Tip: Damp heat is always preferable to dry heat. Hence, a damp hot towel is more effective than a heat mat.

Electrical muscle stimulation (EMS)

Electrical muscle stimulation is sometimes referred to as Estim or NMES (neuromuscular electrical stimulation). These are all the same thing. EMS is sometimes also referred to as TENS (transcutaneous nerve stimulation). Whilst both use the same machine, TENS uses completely different settings to achieve pain relief by stimulating the sensory fibres. EMS is used to reverse or reduce muscle atrophy by stimulating motor fibres.

Mobile units are most commonly used in veterinary physiotherapy (Figure 5.3). EMS machine consists of a small box with a battery and buttons for adjusting the settings and two sets of leads. Each set of leads has a pad at each end. The pads are placed at the top and bottom of the muscle and a current is passed. This causes the muscle to contract. Clipping of the fur and application of an aqueous gel are required to ensure a good contact. The kit comprises two sets of leads, so that two muscle groups can be stimulated at the same time. For instance, one pair of pads could be attached to the quadriceps muscle group and the other to the hamstring group of muscle (Figure 5.4). The muscle can be made to contract at the same time (synchronised mode), in which case the joint will not move, or set to contract alternately (alternate mode), in which case the stifle extends and flexes as each group contracts.

Settings

Mode: Continuous, synchronised or alternate. Switch the unit on by lifting the transparent cover on the top of the machine and turning the two dials to the 1 position

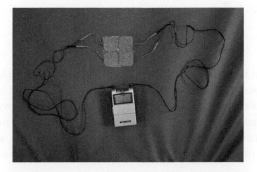

Figure 5.3 The EMS unit consists of a battery-powered control unit with two channels each consisting of a negative and positive lead and two contact pads.

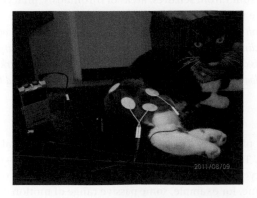

Figure 5.4 An EMS unit being used on a cat with a femoral fracture.

(Figure 5.5(a)). Press the MODE button until the desired sequence is displayed. Continuous mode is used to adjust the milliamp setting to just cause a contraction. The mode should then be switched to synchronised or alternate. Continuous mode is also used in TENS (see below).

Pulse duration or pulse width is the duration of one pulse and is measured in microseconds (µs). Pulse duration between 100 and 400 µs is typically used for muscle building. To adjust the machine, see Figure 5.5(b).

Frequency or pulse rate is the number of pulses per second and is measured in hertz (Hz). A frequency of 25–50 Hz would be typical for muscle stimulation (Figure 5.5(c)).

Time is set for the total running time of each treatment session (Figure 5.5(d)).

Ramp is the length of time that the current is gradually increased or decreased. Ramp-up and ramp-down of 4 seconds would be typical (Figure 5.5(e)).

On/Off cycle is the length of time the current is on or off. On/Off cycle ratio of 1:3 indicates that the current is on for 5 seconds and off for 15 seconds. For weaker muscles, the off time will need to be increased to avoid fatigue (Figure 5.5(f)).

Amplitude. This is measured in milliamps (mA). The higher the mA setting the stronger the contraction as more muscle fibres are recruited. The operator adjusts the mA once the electrodes have been put in place. The mA is gradually increased until a contraction is observed. The mA should not be increased so as to cause discomfort (Figure 5.5(g)).

Each session lasts between 5 and 20 minutes depending on the degree of muscle fatigue.

Indications

EMS is useful when there is, or to prevent, muscle atrophy. It can be used preoperatively as well as post-operatively. It can also be used if the patient is recumbent. The mobile units are inexpensive and can be hired or purchased by owners. The settings can be pre-set by the veterinarian or physiotherapist and the owners shown where to place the pads. The owner then just has to slowly increase mA setting by turning the dial on the top of the unit until a muscle contraction is observed.

Contraindications

Pregnacy, wounds, malignancy, patients with pacemakers, over the site of a laminectomy, patients that suffer from seizures, areas of thrombosis, pharyngeal area, carotid sinus and anywhere that movement is contraindicated.

Tip: The EMS unit can be loaned to owners so that they can carry out the treatment in between visits to the clinic. If the dog has been shaved, for example, for surgery or arthroscopy, the position of the pads can be drawn on the dog's skin with a non-toxic marker pen (Figure 5.6). Alternatively, if the dog has not been shaved, small patches can be clipped to indicate the positioning of the pads.

TENS

The electrodes are placed over the area of pain or the peripheral nerve roots that innervate the area. Typical settings would be: pulse duration, 50–100 µs; frequency, 150 Hz; no on/off cycle and no ramp. The duration of the session will be determined by what is being done, for example, some passive range of motion exercises. Remember that the pain relief at this frequency will only be present when the current passes.

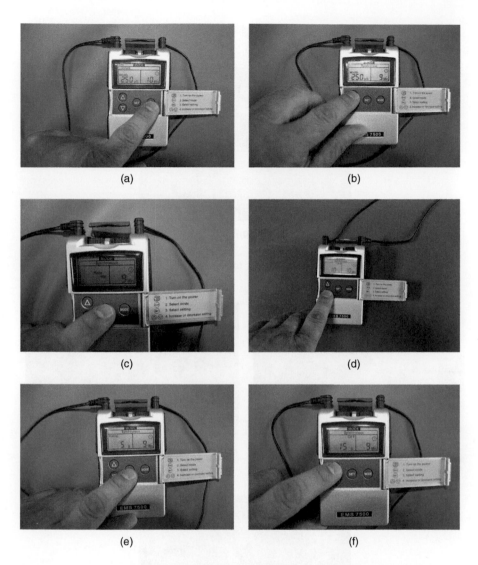

Figure 5.5 (a) Turn on by turning the dials on the top of the machine. Press the MODE button until the desired sequence is displayed. Usually *Synchronised* or *Alternate*. (b) Press the SET button until the *Width* setting is displayed. Use the up and down keys to attain the desired setting, usually between 100 and 400 μs. (c) Press SET button until Rate is displayed. Use the up and down keys to attain the desired setting, usually between 25 and 50 Hz. (d) Press the SET button until the *Time* flashes in the right-hand side screen. Use the up and down keys to select the total number of minutes per treatment session, usually between 5 and 20 minutes. (e) Press the SET button again to reach the Ramp setting. Use the up and down arrows to select the appropriate time, usually 4–8 seconds. (f) Press the SET button to display the ON time. Use the up and down buttons to select the appropriate time, usually 5–10 seconds. Press the SET key again to display the OFF time. Use the up and down keys to select the appropriate time, usually 2–5 times the ON time. (g) Adjust the Amplitude by turning the dials on the top of the machine until a contraction is observed.

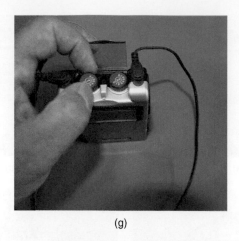

(g)

Figure 5.5   (*continued*)

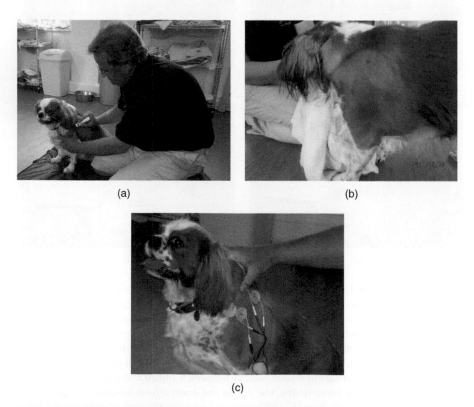

(a)

(b)

(c)

Figure 5.6   If the patient has been shaved, the position of the contact pads can be marked on the skin with a marker pen for the owner.

It has no residual pain-relieving properties. Pain relief by using TENS in the dog is difficult to evaluate.

Laser therapy

Lasers have been used for many years in human physiotherapy and are now beginning to make quite an impact in the veterinary market (Figures 5.7 and 5.8).

Lasers are divided into classes depending on power as follows:

Class	Example	Comments
Class 1	CD player	No risk to tissues
Class 2 (<1 mW)	Laser pointer	Little threat of eye damage
Class 3a (1–5 mW)	Visible light therapy machines	Threat of eye damage
Class 3b (5–500 mW)	Non-visible therapy machines	Can cause eye damage
Class 4 (>500 mW)	Surgical and rehab machines	High risk of tissue damage, blinding and burning

Penetration is determined by wavelength. Wavelength is predetermined in each machine. Therapeutic wavelength range is 600–940 nm. Some of the newer Class 4

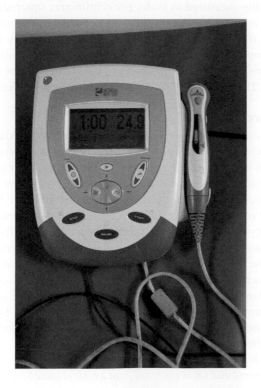

Figure 5.7   A typical Class 3b laser and probe.

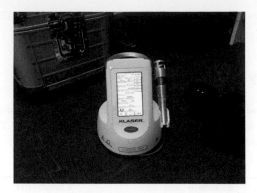

Figure 5.8   An example of a Class 4 laser. These machines have 10–20 times the power of a Class 3b laser. Safety goggles must be worn.

lasers have beams of multiple wavelengths (K-Laser Cube). Absorption will occur at various levels as the beam passes through different tissues. This is an important factor when selecting the dosage to be delivered (see Dosage).

Lasers deliver energy (joules) that depends on the power (watts) of the laser and the time the laser is on. Class 3b lasers only have up to 500 mW of power. The laser probe can be directed at the target joint or tissue and held in place while the dosage is delivered (normally measured in joules per centimetres squared). A Class 4 laser produces so much energy that the head has to be held away from the patient and constantly moved in order to prevent burning. Health and safety for Class 4 lasers requires that all people in the room where lasers are used must wear protective goggles, the patient should be hooded, the doors to the room must be locked or a clear NO ENTRY LASER THERAPY IN PROGRESS sign must be displayed.

Effects of lasers

Therapeutic lasers cause an increase in cell metabolic rate by affecting part of Kreb's Cycle in the mitochondria. The result is an increase in ATP production and cell metabolic rate. This increase in cell metabolic rate results in faster production of the material the cell manufactures, for example, fibroblast produce more collagen and chondrocytes produce more cartilage matrix. There is also evidence that laser therapy can enhance nerve recovery. Lasers also decrease the number of microorganisms, by increasing lymphocyte production, which can have a dramatic effect on granulating wounds and contaminated/infected areas, for example, otitis externa.

Lasers also cause the local release of nitrous oxide, which causes vasodilation. Therefore, lasers increase the blood supply to an area. Lasers also reduce the production of prostaglandins and Cox-2 (cyclo-oxygenase coenzyme-2) in the synovial membrane and synovial fluid and in so doing reduce joint pain. Lasers also reduce pain by reducing nerve firing at neuromuscular junctions. Lasers also cause the release of endorphins that enhance pain relief.

Tip: It is always better to laser an animal when it is on the ground. Many dogs will fall asleep whilst being lasered and could easily fall from a table (Figure 5.9).

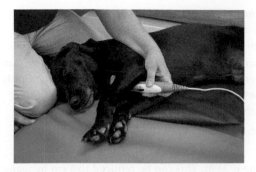

Figure 5.9   Patients often fall asleep while being lasered.

Dosage

Most lasers come with pre-set dosages for different tissues and whether the injury is acute or chronic. As a guide, acute injuries require 3–5 j/cm², subacute injuries 7–10 j/cm² and chronic injuries 12–24 j/cm². As mentioned earlier, the beam will be subject to absorption as it passes through various tissues and this absorption will need to be taken into account when deciding on settings.

Coat/Skin colour

Dark coats/skin will absorb more energy whereas light coats/skin cause more scatter of the beam. The end result is that the amount of energy required is approximately the same.

Calculating the dosage

$1\,j = 1$ watt $\times 1$ second.

Irradiation time in seconds $= (\{D \times A\}/P) \times \{1 + d\}$.

$D =$ desired dose at target tissue (joules/cm²).

$A =$ Area of target tissue in cm².

$P =$ Power of laser in Watts.

$d =$ Depth of target tissue.

Therefore, for a Class 3b laser with a 500 mW (0.5 W) head treating a Labrador with stifle OA, the equation is as follows:

Desired dose at the stifle, 15 j/cm².

Treating around the joint line to lateral, cranial and medial aspects, target area would be 15 cm².

Power is 0.5 W.

Depth of target tissue, d, is 0.5 cm.

Irradiation time $= (\{15 \times 15\}/0.5) \times \{1 + 0.5\} = 675$ seconds $= 11$ minutes 15 seconds.

If you laser at 10 points around the stifle, this equates to 67.5 seconds per point.

Tip: If using a Class 3b laser and treating a deep tissue or joint, gently push the laser head into the patient whilst aiming at the target to reduce the distance the beam has to travel (depth). This will reduce the time needed to deliver the correct amount of energy.

Here is another example of a dosage calculation for treating a Labrador with hip OA using a Class 3b laser with a 500 mW head and a Class 4 laser with a 5 W head.

For the Class 3b laser:

Desired dose at target tissue, 20 j/cm^2.

Area of target tissue, 15 cm^2.

Power $= 0.5$ W.

Depth of target tissue is 3 cm. This can be reduced to 1 cm by using the tip above.

Irradiation time $= (\{20 \times 15\}/0.5) \times \{1 + 1\} = 1200$ seconds or 20 minutes.

If you laser at 15 points around the hip, this equates to 80 seconds per point.

Using a 5 W Class 4 laser to treat the same dog.

Desired dosage, 20 j/cm^2.

Area of target tissue, 15 cm^2.

Power $= 5$ W.

Depth $= 4$ cm (Class 4 laser must be held approximately 1 cm above the skin and moved constantly to avoid burning).

Irradiation time $= (\{20 \times 15\}/) \times (1 + 4) = 300$ seconds $= 5$ minutes.

Setting the laser

Class 3b. Each machine will differ, but wavelength and power are predetermined on the machine. The time setting is adjusted to deliver the calculated dose.

Most of the *Class 4* lasers available in the veterinary market have their own pre-installed programs. These work out the dosage to be delivered taking into account coat colour, weight of animal, area to be lasered and stage of healing, for example, acute, subacute or chronic. The increased power of these machines does mean significantly reduced treatment times. However, the laser head is held about 1 cm above the treatment area and is constantly moved to avoid overheating/burning of the skin. This is a particular problem with dark coated dogs that absorb more energy.

Implants

Lasers are safe to use over implants composed of metal, plastic or cement. The implants will not warm up as laser therapy uses light (phototherapy) and not heat therapy. However, the metal implants will absorb the entire laser light and prevent penetration to deeper tissues. Therefore, it is better to laser from the other side of the leg, for example, lasering from the lateral side of a TPLO procedure. Remember dosage will have to be adjusted because of the greater depth of target tissue.

Lasers can be used in patients with cardiac disease and areas of impaired circulation. They can also be used in patients with electronic devices, for example, pacemakers.

Lasers can also be used on acupuncture points.

Protocols: Acute or post-operative injuries should be treated every other day, subacute injuries twice weekly. With chronic conditions, such as osteoarthritis, treatments may start off at weekly and then gradually extend to monthly as they progress.

Contraindications

Lasers should not be used in dogs with malignancy. Other contraindications are pregnancy, around the eye or carotid sinus, photosensitisation and bleeding disorders.

Therapeutic ultrasound

Therapeutic ultrasound machines differ from diagnostic ultrasound machines (Figure 5.10). It is not possible to use a diagnostic ultrasound as a therapeutic ultrasound and vice versa. Therapeutic ultrasound uses very high-frequency sound waves that are converted to kinetic energy as the waves move through the tissues. Therapeutic ultrasound is most effective in high-protein tissues, such as ligaments.

The effects of therapeutic ultrasound are divided into thermal and non-thermal. Thermal effects promote blood flow to an area, reduce pain and increase joint- and soft-tissue flexibility. This is similar to superficial heating, but penetrates much deeper. Non-thermal effects are acoustic streaming and cavitation. Acoustic streaming results from the small pressure waves in the interstitial fluid. Cavitation results from compression and expansion of gas bubbles in the interstitial fluid. Both these are thought to affect cell membrane permeability.

Most therapeutic ultrasound machines have two settings: 1 and 3 MHz. The 1 MHz setting is used for deeper tissues and will penetrate to a depth of 2–5 cm. The 3 MHz setting is used for more superficial tissues as it only penetrates up to 1–2 cm.

Continuous mode

In continuous mode, the energy stream is constantly on. This is used when the thermal effect is desired (i.e. heating).

Pulsed mode

In the pulsed mode, the energy stream is turned on and off. The duty cycle usually ranges from 5% to 50%, that is, the energy stream is on for 5% to 50% of the time. This mode is used when the non-thermal effects are desired, and is particularly useful when treating tendon lesions as it helps break down adhesions between the tendon and its sheath (Figure 5.11).

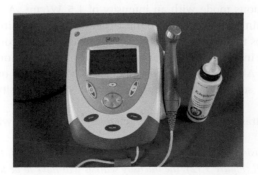

Figure 5.10   An example of a therapeutic ultrasound machine.

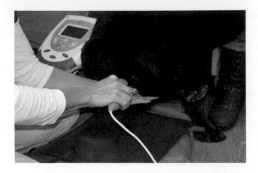

Figure 5.11   Pulsed ultrasound being used on Achilles tendinopathy to try to break down adhesions between the tendon and its sheath.

Intensity

This is measured in Watts/cm^2. Settings usually range from 0.1 to 3.0 W/cm^2. The tissue being treated will determine the intensity setting, its depth and the mode selected.

Time

Treatment times are normally between 5 and 10 minutes depending on size of animal and depth of tissue.

It is important that there is an air-free contact between the skin and the probe as ultrasound will not pass through air. Shaving helps to reduce air bubbles forming between the hairs of the coat, which owners often see as a retrograde step in recovery. Copious use of ultrasound gel may negate the need to shave. Alternatively, the patient can be treated with the target area under water in an underwater treadmill if available or in a bucket of water if the area is below the hock or carpus. If this technique is used, the intensity and time settings will have to be increased.

Normally the treatment area is about 2–3 times the size of the probe head. The transducer head is moved slowly and evenly over the target area for the duration of the treatment.

Examples

To warm the deep gluteal muscles on a German Shepherd dog, 1 MHz would be selected in continuous mode with an intensity of 1.5 W/cm^2. A typical treatment time would be 7 minutes. Copious amounts of gel would be required.

To treat a biceps tendonitis in a Labrador Retriever, 3 MHz would be selected in pulsed mode 50%, intensity 0.8 W/cm^2 for 6 minutes. Again copious amounts of gel would be needed. Alternatively, the treatment could be carried out in the UWTM in which case the settings would be adjusted to 1 MHz, intensity 1.5 W/cm^2 for 7.5 minutes.

Therapeutic ultrasound machines are relatively inexpensive when compared to lasers.

Tip: If you are using the ultrasound on an area whilst submerged, for example, in the underwater treadmill (Figure 5.12), the intensity settings will have to be increased by at least 0.5 W/cm^2, especially if the ultrasound is being used in continuous mode as the water has a cooling effect on the tissues.

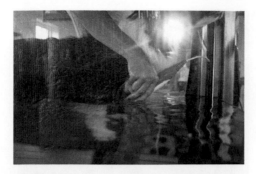

Figure 5.12   Ultrasounding a dog in the underwater treadmill.

Pulsed electromagnetic field therapy (PEMFT)

This is sometimes referred to as short wave or diathermy short wave. The latter of these terms is confusing as no heat is involved. At higher power levels (over 5 W), there can be some thermal effects. There is little or no scientific evidence to support the use of static magnets as therapeutic agents despite their popularity. However, there is scientific evidence emerging to support the use of strong electromagnetic fields that are pulsed.

Theory

The exact mechanism of action is not yet known. It has been suggested that PEMFT interferes with nerve transmission in small unmyelinated nerve, for example, C fibres (pain) by changing resting cell membrane potentials. Also in damaged tissue, there is a leakage of potassium from within cells into the interstitial tissues. This again alters the resting cell membrane potential. It is thought that PEMFT can increase ion exchange in areas of damage. Ion exchange is responsible for oxygen utilisation within the cell.

The system consists of a mat that contains a wire coil and a control box (Figure 5.13).

Electric current is passed through the wire coil which produces a three-dimensional magnetic field around the coil. The current is switched on and off (pulsed) very rapidly. This background pulse may then have an interference pulse applied. Settings vary from manufacturer and model. The action of PEMFT is aimed at blocking pain transmission or increasing oxygen utilisation in areas of damage. The latter is thought to result in an increased blood supply to areas of damage.

The area to be treated is positioned so as to be in the magnetic field. This may just involve lying on the mat or wearing the coat. Treatment times are up to 20 minutes. The effects of PEMFT will last for approximately 6 hours after treatment. Treatment can be repeated twice daily.

PEMFT units are inexpensive and maybe considered for owners to buy for treating their animals at home.

Contraindications

Make sure that neither the dog nor the owner has a pacemaker. The magnetic field with PEMFT is sufficient to interfere with the functioning of these

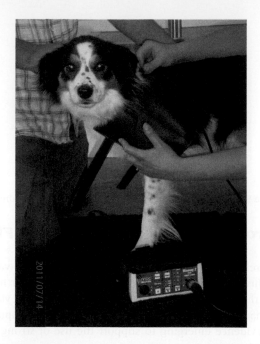

Figure 5.13   Pulsed electromagnetic field therapy mat on a patient's shoulder.

machines. Pregnancy and malignancy are also contraindicated. If the owner is pregnant, has a pacemaker or malignancy, they should be at least 3 m away or in another room.

Extracorporeal shockwave therapy (ESWT)

Extracorporeal shockwave therapy (ESWT) does not involve electrical shocks. It is sometimes referred to as high-energy pressure therapy. It uses a very short burst of very high-energy waves or pulses to create large sudden changes in pressure. Examples of such large rapid changes in pressure in nature would be supersonic aircraft boom, explosions and lightening. It is called extracorporeal as the pressure change is generated outside the patient's body. ESWT penetrates deeper than any other modality.

The rapid high change in pressure is produced by three different methods.

1 Electrohydraulic (PulseVet VersaTron)

A high-voltage electric current is passed across a spark gap in a water-filled container. This produces a vapourisation bubble that expands and immediately collapses. A high-energy pressure wave is the result. This is then focused using a reflector. This method produces the highest peak pressure in the shortest time (Figure 5.14). Two heads or trodes are supplied. Each trode comes preloaded with several thousand shocks. Once the shocks have been used up, the trodes are returned to the manufacturer for recharging.

2 Electromagnetic (Storz Minilith)

A high voltage is applied to electromagnetic coil. This produces changes in pressure similar to the effect of a loud speaker. This produces a pressure change of about one-third of the electrohydraulic machine.

3 Piezoelectric (Wolf PiezoSon, Chattanooga Shockwave)

Submerged piezoelectric crystals are stimulated with high-frequency electrical impulses. This creates ultrasonic vibrations that result in a shockwave. This produces the smallest change in pressure (Figure 5.15). The head comes with 1 million shocks preloaded.

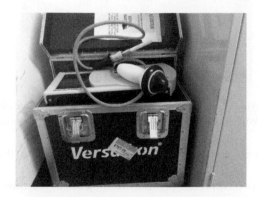

Figure 5.14 An example of a hydroelectric shockwave machine. PulseVet.

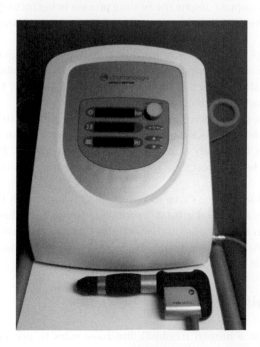

Figure 5.15 An example of a Piezoelectric shockwave. Chattanooga.

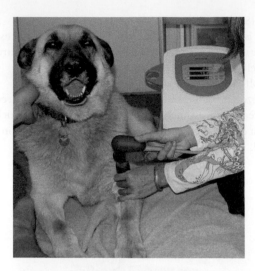

Figure 5.16   A dog having Piezoelectric shockwave applied to an arthritic elbow. No sedation is required in this case. With hydroelectric shockwave, the patient would have needed sedation.

Electrohydraulic shockwave penetrates the deepest, but is also the most expensive machine.

ESWT works in two ways. The first is by causing micro-fractures in the target tissue be it bone or soft tissue. These micro-fractures cause a new wave of inflammation. ESWT is particularly useful in treating tendons and ligaments where often the inflammatory process has stopped despite the healing process being incomplete. ESWT also stimulates the production of angiogenic growth factors that promote increased blood supply to the area.

The second way ESWT works is as the shockwave passes through the tissues, there is a void behind the wave. Cavitation bubbles form in this void. When the cavitation bubbles hit a hard surface, they collapse. As the bubbles collapse, they break down mineral deposits, such as calcified nodules in tendons.

Electrohydraulic shockwave is uncomfortable for the patient, and hence sedation is required. Piezoelectric shockwave can be carried out without sedation. Up to three treatments at fortnightly intervals is the normal protocol. In dogs, ESWT is particularly useful for the treatment of shoulder tendinopathies (Figure 5.16) (see Chapter 8).

A gel is applied to the dog's coat to ensure good contact with the head (trode). Different trode sizes are available for different target areas. Typical settings for shoulder tendinopathy in a Labrador would be 800–2000 shocks per treatment depending on type of ESWT machine. The treatment time is only a few minutes. Occasionally, dogs may feel a little discomfort for 48 hours after treatment.

Land treadmill

These are similar to a human treadmill, but have sides to prevent the dog from jumping off (Figure 5.17). Land treadmills are good for strengthening, endurance and cardiovascular fitness. Most are able to incline/decline that also allows increased

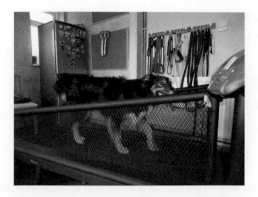

Figure 5.17   A dog on a land treadmill. Note the retaining sides.

weight distribution to back/front legs accordingly. Care must be taken when using the incline/decline not to exacerbate or over load pathological conditions such as hip OA or carpal hyperextension.

Hydrotherapy

In recent years, hydrotherapy has become well established as a treatment option for animals. Hydrotherapy works in several different ways to facilitate a return to normal function.

Water temperature
The water temperature for hydrotherapy, be it a pool or underwater treadmill, is between 29 and 32 °C. This has the effect of warming and increasing blood supply to the submerged tissues as well as relaxing the patient. It provides an excellent environment for doing therapeutic exercises that may be difficult on land. The warm water also produces sensory stimulation that is important in spinal cases.

Buoyancy
The more of the body that is submerged, the less weight will be taken through the joints. This allows painful joints to move more easily due to reduced loading.

Hydrostatic effect
The hydrostatic effect is the pressure the water puts on the parts of the body that are submerged. The hydrostatic effect will help reduce swelling and venous congestion in the sub-chondral bone that has been cited as a major cause of pain in arthritic joints.

Tip: Older arthritic dogs may not be keen to walk in the UWTM or swim. However, these dogs still benefit from just standing in the warm water and taking advantage of the hydrostatic effect (Figure 5.18).

Viscosity
Water viscosity provides resistance to movement. This is an extremely good way to help rebuild muscle. Resistance can be further increased by the use of water jets. The

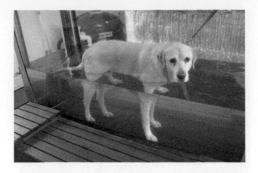

Figure 5.18   An old dog with elbow and hip osteoarthritis standing in water to take advantage of the hydrostatic effect and warmth of the water.

resistance can also be useful to correct gait abnormalities such as the swaggering gait with hip dysplasia.

Support

The water offers support to the body that it would not experience on land. This is useful for the neurological patient who may be uncoordinated and liable to falling. The water will support the body and slow down the fall. This allows the patient to take more time to correct the incoordination and avoid falling.

Pool versus underwater treadmill (UWTM)

Both pools and UWTM have advantages and disadvantages. Pools that have sub-merged platforms (Figure 5.19) allow for a greater range of treatment protocols than pools that just have an entry and exit ramp. Simply, swimming will help cardiovas-cular fitness, weight loss and endurance better than the UWTM. Care must also be exercised when swimming an acute front leg lameness. The idea that swimming can do no harm is incorrect.

For rehabilitation, the UWTM offers far more variation and control. The depth of water and speed of the belt can be carefully controlled. Monitoring of leg movement

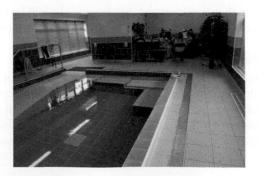

Figure 5.19   An example of a pool with submerged platforms that allow therapeutic exercises to be conducted in the warm and stimulating water environment.

and observation of the patient from the front, back, both sides and above are possible with the UWTM (Figure 5.20(a)–(d)) On some machines, individual profiles can be recorded that allows progress to be monitored. Also, in the UWTM, the patient is weight bearing. The pushing of the leg through the water while walking tends to build muscle quicker than by swimming (Figure 5.21). The UWTM also offers hydrotherapy to certain breeds where swimming could pose significant problems (e.g. Bassett Hound).

Tip: If only one side of the treadmill can be accessed, a mirror can be placed on the far side to view the dog walking. In addition, measuring strips are available for the outside of the tank so that various comparisons of stride length can be recorded.

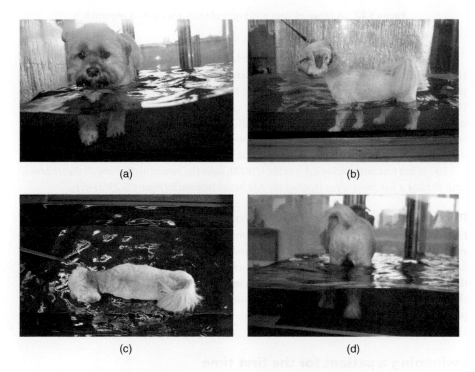

(a)   (b)

(c)   (d)

Figure 5.20   (a)–(d) The UWTM allows the dog to be observed moving from the front, both sides, above and behind.

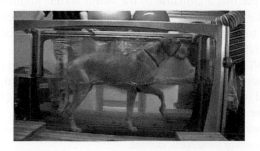

Figure 5.21   The viscosity of water provides resistance that helps build muscle.

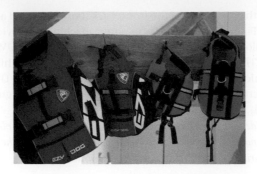

Figure 5.22   A range of sizes and types of buoyancy aids is required.

With both pool and UWTM, a good selection of floatation vests and harnesses (Figure 5.22) is required as well as toys and treats. Patients should be introduced very gradually to hydrotherapy schedules. For example, for most patients using the UWTM for the first time, the session may only last 2 minutes. Gradually build this up to 10–20 minutes. Depth can also be adjusted. If possible, fill the tank so that the water covers the joint(s) being treated. However, if the water level is very high, the dog will attempt to swim which may not be desired.

Tip: When first introducing a dog to the UWTM, have the owner walk through the treadmill with the dog a few times, even treating the dog in the treadmill (Figure 5.23(a)–(c)).

Putting a patient in the UWTM for the first time

Encourage the owner to go to the head end and tempt with treats and toys. Start with the water just above the dog's feet and at a slow speed until the dog becomes accustomed to walking on a moving platform (1–2 minutes). The water level can be then be increased as the dog becomes acclimatised to the UWTM. The first session should last not more than 4 minutes in total. The first few times in the UWTM, the patient will be very tired after the session. *Do not overwork weak or fatigued muscles!* (Figures 5.24(a)–(d)).

Swimming a patient for the first time

Make sure the patient is fitted with a suitable buoyancy aid. A therapist should accompany the dog into the pool (Figure 5.25). Ideally, entry should be via a ramp (Figure 5.26). Let the dog acclimatise to the warm water. Additional support from the therapist will be required if the dog is unable to support itself with a paddling action. NEVER try to support a patient from poolside with a metal pole attached to the harness and no therapist in the water.

As with the UWTM, dogs will tire quickly the first few times in the pool. Sessions should again be restricted to just a few minutes of assisted swimming. Swim time is gradually increased with intervals for rest. Manual therapies (see Chapter 6) can also be carried out in the stimulating warm environment.

Tip: When swimming or doing manual therapies in a pool, have an abacus poolside to count the number of laps or sets of therapeutic exercise.

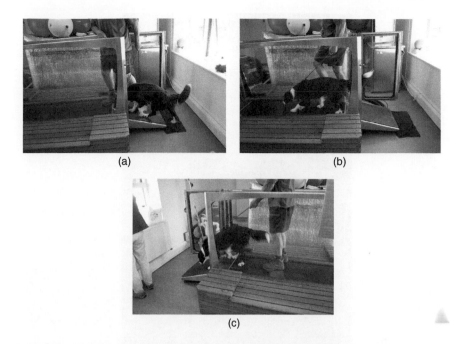

Figure 5.23 (a)–(c) Familiarise the dog to the treadmill by having the owner walk the dog through the treadmill several times before closing the doors.

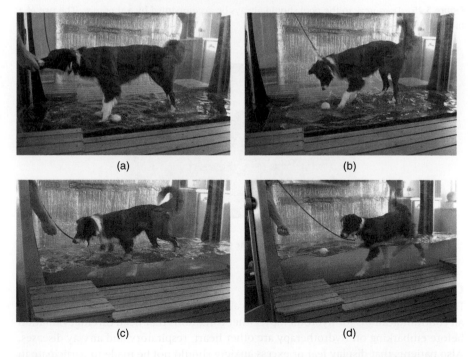

Figure 5.24 (a) Treats and toys are used to encourage the dogs to walk in the UWTM. (b)–(d) The water level can be gradually increased as the dog acclimatises to the UWTM. Start at foot height, then hock height and then stifle height. Not more than 1 minute at each height for a novice dog.

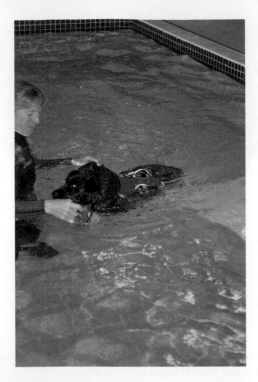

Figure 5.25   Dogs new to the pool should always be accompanied by a therapist. The use of a metal pole from poolside is unacceptable.

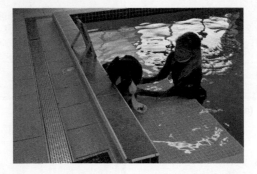

Figure 5.26   Entry and exit from the pool should ideally be by a ramp.

Contraindications

Heart failure, open wounds, healing surgical wounds, skin disease and diarrhoea are all contraindications for hydrotherapy. Other conditions that need careful evaluation before embarking on hydrotherapy are other heart, respiratory and airway diseases. Also patients that display fear or excess anxiety should not be made to participate in hydrotherapy.

CHAPTER 6

Manual therapies

Manual therapy is an umbrella term used for the therapeutic handling techniques covering numerous soft-tissue techniques including massage, passive movements and joint mobilisations. All manual therapy techniques affect joint movement either directly or indirectly by movement of the soft tissues and thus moving the joints. The term massage is the movement of the soft tissue and covers a number of light to deep touch techniques. These include kneading, effleurage, myofascial release, trigger point release and transverse friction massage. Joint mobilisations can be performed on peripheral and vertebral joints covering dorsoventral pressures on the facet joints of the spine, distraction or traction, accessory movements and passive movements.

When performing manual techniques, it is important that the therapist is aware of how they perform them in their own manner. Manual techniques should not be rushed as this will make the dog tense and becomes counterproductive. The therapist also needs to be calm in his/her manner and be able to put the animal and owner at ease.

Massage

Massage is often considered as part of the treatment in animal physiotherapy and can be used as a way of preparing the soft tissues for other treatments. The release of tight musculature will prepare the body for passive joint stretching and can, therefore, increase the range of movement that can be achieved. Massage not only acts on muscle and fascial systems, but also the nervous and circulatory systems. However, function cannot be restored through massage alone. The same is true of joint mobilisation; abnormal muscle tone and tension will occur following abnormal movement patterns. Once mobility is restored in a joint, the movement pattern will not be corrected until the muscle tightness and imbalance are addressed and vice versa. The muscle will not function normally if the joints they move remain restricted.

Massage is also a useful tool for physiotherapists to improve their palpation skills, distinguishing between normal and abnormal tones, atrophy and hypertrophy, fibrous thickenings and tissue swelling.

Practical Physiotherapy for Small Animal Practice, First Edition.
Edited by David Prydie and Isobel Hewitt.
© 2015 John Wiley & Sons, Ltd. Published 2015 by John Wiley & Sons, Ltd.
Companion Website: www.wiley.com/go/practical-physiotherapy-for-small-animals

Effects of massage

Reduce stress

The activation of sensory nerves during massage can produce a soothing effect (depending on the technique used and the pressure applied during the techniques). If slow rhythmical massage is used, relaxation and well-being are induced, which can aid recovery.

Reduce ACTH production

Massage increases oxytocin levels, which counteracts the release of ACTH.

Lymphatics

Following acute injury, tissue fluid can leak out of the blood vessels and accumulate in the tissue spaces. If the circulatory system is compromised and therefore unable to remove the fluid, massage can then be effective to remove the fluid. The flow of lymph in the lymphatic system can be in any direction, but the force from muscle contraction or movement and gravity usually controls the flow. The mechanical pressure placed on the tissue spaces by massage will aid the movement of the tissue fluid or lymph back into the circulatory system.

Circulation

Massage affects vasomotor nerves and stimulates vasodilation. This can be seen on the skin as 'pinkness' or erythema where the skin is visible. The mechanical movement of the massage strokes can move blood in the veins and increase arterial flow. An increase in blood flow will aid recovery through increased nutrition and oxygen.

Muscle spindles

These monitor the changes in muscle length and can control muscle stretch along with the Golgi tendon organs. The muscle spindles contain stretch receptors that respond to either slow, sustained or rapid stretch of the muscle fibres. The Golgi tendon organs will monitor dynamic and static tension changes in tendon fibres. They have a protective inhibitory role via the reflex arcs of muscles and also have a role in the control of muscle tone. The muscle spindles have a facilitatory reflex arc that will contract muscle fibres in opposition to the original stretch. The muscles spindles can respond to velocity of stretch, such as a patella reflex, or a prolonged stretch. The Golgi tendon organs are activated after 6 seconds of stretching and will cause a reflex relaxation. Knowledge of how the muscle spindles and Golgi tendon organs are stimulated will influence our handling skills, especially when performing passive movements.

Effect on muscle tone

Massage reduces muscle spasm and can aid recovery of muscles following vigorous exercise, through the increase in circulation that will remove waste materials such as lactic acid. The extensibility and elasticity of muscles is enhanced by massage and can prevent formation of fibrous adhesions between muscles and fascia.

Pain

Massage stimulates a^δ (delta) fibres in the skin. These give pain relief through the pain gate mechanism. The a^δ fibres are faster acting than the C fibres, therefore can 'close the gate' to pain.

Increased stretch in connective tissue

The movement and stretch of the collagen fibres within connective tissue can loosen adherent structures, for example, scars and tendons bound down within their sheaths.

Improve performance in the working dog

Massage can be used to maintain the condition of muscles. In addition, massage before exercise can increase the blood flow to the muscles helping them to work more efficiently.

Indications for massage

Behaviour
Chronic orthopaedic problems
Post operation
Muscle atrophy
Improve lymph and blood flow
Reduce pain
Reduce scar formation

Contraindications

Because of the effects of increased blood flow, there are a number of absolute contraindications to massage as follows: malignant tumours; advanced disease of the blood vessels, either atherosclerosis or arteriosclerosis; thrombosis; shock; infectious diseases such as fever and temperament of the animal (aggressive).

There are also local contraindications and precautions to massage: areas of acute inflammation; areas of haemorrhage and active haematoma (although gentle massage can later help to break down and disperse haematoma); sites of unstable fractures; open skin wounds, where there is infection of the skin; skin that is in poor condition or sensitive and may bruise easily; long-term steroid treatment, which may leave skin weakened and more susceptible to damage.

Deep transverse friction massage is also contraindicated when there is calcification or ossification of the soft tissues and should not be used on nerve tissue and inflamed bursae.

Care should also be taken for patients with heart, liver and kidney problems.

Types of massage
Stroking in direction of hair

This is often used as an introductory or preparatory technique as it will give the therapist a chance to assess the tension/tone of the tissue enabling him/her to select the most appropriate technique for the main treatment. It can be very useful to calm an anxious animal and will help relax excessive muscle spasm. It can be a deep or superficial stroke, which is performed by using the hands or finger pads. The speed of the strokes will determine the effect; slow will produce a soothing effect and quick will produce stimulation. It directly affects the sensory nerve fibres and produces a sedative or stimulated feeling. Stroking will also result in the release of a histamine-like

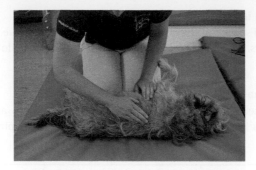

Figure 6.1   *Stroking technique.* Place hands or finger pads on the surface of the animal and stroke in the direction of the hair.

chemical that can cause dilation of capillaries preparing for an increase in blood flow to the tissue from other techniques (Figure 6.1).

Effleurage

Effleurage is where the hands are moulded around the body part to be massaged and the strokes are applied in the direction of venous and lymphatic flow. When effleurage is applied to a leg the direction of strokes will be distal to proximal. The desired effect is to move the fluid towards the lymph nodes at the proximal end of the leg. The pressure needs to be even throughout the leg, but be careful to avoid any bony prominences. This technique can be stimulatory or sedative depending on the rate and depth applied. Effleurage has mechanical, nervous and chemical effects on the body. The mechanical effect is directly on the venous system, increasing the return of blood and lymph through direct stimulation of the vessels. It will also mobilise the superficial soft tissues. Deep effleurage will stimulate the axon reflex causing arteriole dilation, and the release of a histamine-like substance also causes capillary dilation (Figure 6.2).

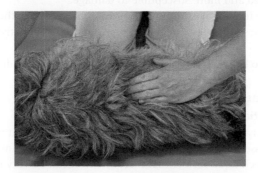

Figure 6.2   *Effleurage technique.* Place the hands on the animal and mould around the body part to be massaged. Apply the strokes in the direction of venous and lymphatic flow.

Petrissage

Petrissage is a term for a group of techniques that can be referred to as 'pressure' manipulations used on muscles and soft tissue. They can be transverse or longitudinal mobilisations that are particularly useful for softening muscles that have become chronically tight as a result of chronically stiff joints.

Kneading

This technique can be performed using palm/finger or thumb pads depending on the size of the area to be treated. If the technique is to be used in an oedematous area, then 'squeeze' kneading can be used. If a large animal is being treated, then 're-enforced kneading' can be used where one hand is placed on top of the other. The important point of the technique is that the muscles or soft tissue is pressed inwards and upwards, squeezed and compressed then released in a circular movement. The direction of the motion should be towards the heart. When treating a leg, the hands are usually placed on opposite sides; if treating the spine, then the hands are placed on either side of the spinal column and the area is treated with the hands working alternatively and rhythmically. As the motion is completed, the hands glide slightly cranially until the area to be treated is completed (Figure 6.3).

Picking-up

This technique is where the hands are placed flat onto the body and the tissues are grasped, lifted, squeezed and released. Care must be taken to keep the heel of the hand in contact with the tissues and flex the metacarpo-phalangeal joints (keeping the fingers straight) throughout the technique. On larger areas, the hands work alternatively and on smaller animals or muscle groups, one hand can be used or finger and thumb pad grasping, but this must be done very carefully and gently (Figure 6.4).

Wringing

This technique uses the same grasp as the picking-up technique, but once the tissues are grasped, they are squeezed alternately between the finger of one hand and the thenar eminence of the other hand (Figure 6.5).

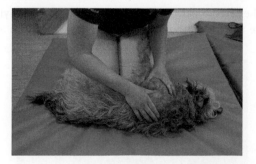

Figure 6.3 *Kneading technique.* Use the palm of the hand/finger or thumb pads depending on the size of area to be treated and press the muscle/soft tissue inwards and upwards, squeeze and compress, then release in one circular movement.

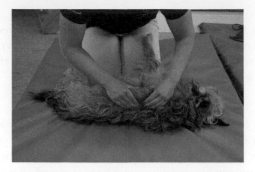

Figure 6.4 *Picking-up technique.* Place the hands flat onto the animal and grasp the tissues, then lift, squeeze and release in one fluid movement.

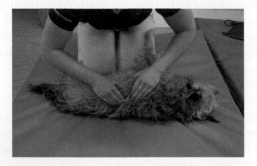

Figure 6.5 *Wringing technique.* Place the hands flat onto the animal and grasp the tissues with the same hold as picking–up, but once the tissues are grasped, squeeze alternately between the finger of one hand and the thenar eminence of the other hand.

Skin rolling

This technique is where the hands are placed flat on the tissues and then the fingers pads draw the tissues back towards the thumbs which in turn roll forwards (Figure 6.6).

The mechanical effects of petrissage are to assist venous and lymphatic flow and mobilise connective tissue and skin. The nervous effect depends again on how the

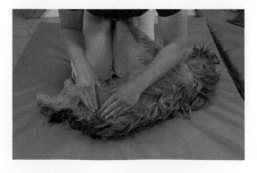

Figure 6.6 *Skin rolling technique.* Place the hands flat on the animal's body and then use the finger pads draw the tissues back towards the thumbs, which in turn roll forwards.

techniques are performed: vigorous will induce vasodilation; brisk and rhythmical are invigorating and slow, deep and rhythmical will reduce spasm and cause relaxation.

Tapotement

This is a term used for techniques that are used to stimulate by striking the body and are meant to be invigorating. These have to be performed carefully with flexible wrists, because if the wrists are locked, they can produce discomfort and would be likely to upset the animal (and owner). In using these techniques, it is also important to explain them carefully to the owner and maybe demonstrate them on the owner first, as to them it may appear that you are hitting the animal.

Clapping/percussion/coupage

This technique is where the hands are cupped and they strike the body alternately. The wrists are flexed and extended to produce the strike with the forearms pronated. The movement at the wrists is soft and rhythmical. The clap will produce a deep hollow sound, not a slapping sound, if performed correctly (Figure 6.7).

Hacking

This technique is where the ulnar borders of the hands and fingers strike the body alternately. The wrists are slightly extended and the strike is produced by pronation and supination of the forearms (Figure 6.8).

These techniques (especially clapping) are mainly used to aid the removal of lung secretions and are best performed when the patient is lying with gravity assisting the drainage of the secretions (a postural drainage position). Clapping can also cause vasodilation and may also elicit the stretch reflex.

Shaking and vibrations

These techniques are again commonly used in respiratory medicine to manually assist the removal of secretions from the lungs. Vibrations can also be useful in neurological conditions where they can facilitate voluntary contractions of severely weakened muscles. They can be more comfortable than clapping and can be more appropriate for animals (and owners) who would not tolerate clapping.

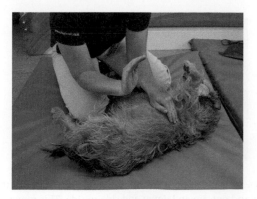

Figure 6.7 *Clapping technique.* Gently cup the hands and strike the body alternately by flexing and extending the wrists.

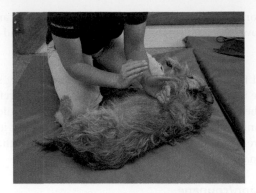

Figure 6.8 *Hacking technique.* Allow the fingers to flex slightly at the metacarpo-phalangeal joints and use the ulnar borders of the hands and fingers strike the body alternately. The strike is produced by the pronation and supination of the wrists.

The technique for these is essentially the same but shaking is a much coarser movement than vibrations. The hands are placed on opposite sides of the lung or area to be treated, and moved in and out, up and down and side to side. A vibration is a fine tremor transmitted through the hands. These techniques can also be performed one-handed if required. The mechanical effect is to displace fluids/secretions, and gases within the lings. This will be more effective if used in conjunction with positioning. Vibrations can be applied slowly and deeply producing a sedative effect on the nervous system. They can produce inhibition of the nervous system which in turn can reduce tension in chronically tight muscles and also may affect the autonomic nervous system (Figure 6.9).

Frictional or Cyriax

These also can be referred to as deep transverse frictions or circular frictions. They are small, deep movements that are localised to the area of treatment. The technique uses either the finger or thumb pads in a transverse or circular motion on the muscle,

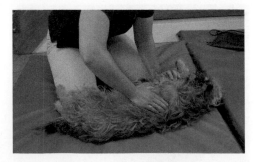

Figure 6.9 *Vibrations technique.* The hands are placed on opposite sides of the lung or area to be treated and moved in and out, up and down and side to side. This movement is a fine tremor transmitted through the hands.

tendon or ligament to be treated. Circular frictions can be very useful on muscular lesions and the pressure applied is progressively increased. On tendon and ligamentous lesion, the preferred technique would be transverse frictions where the finger or thumb is rolled to and fro over the lesion. Before performing frictions, it is important that the patient is as relaxed as possible to allow the technique to penetrate as deeply as you require.

There are a number of different hand/finger positions that can be used when performing frictions and it is useful to try these different techniques to find the one that is most comfortable for you. The size of the lesion or size of the animal may also be a factor in choosing which position works for you.

- Crossing your middle finger over the index finger (Figure 6.10).
- Crossing the index finger over the middle finger (Figure 6.11).
- Two finger pads working side by side across a tendon (Figure 6.12).
- The thumb pad with the distal interphalangeal joint flexed (Figure 6.13).

When applying the friction, care must be taken to not just roll the finger over the skin as this will cause irritation but the skin and subcutaneous tissue must be moved over the muscle, ligament or tendon to produce the desired effect. The pressure applied to the area is directly related to the depth of the lesion from the skin

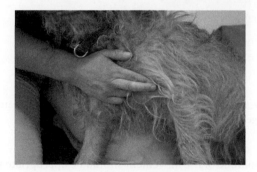

Figure 6.10 *Friction technique.* Place your fingers on the lesion to be treated and cross the middle finger over the index finger and draw the fingers forwards and backwards over the lesion.

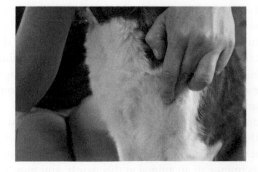

Figure 6.11 *Friction technique.* Place your fingers on the lesion to be treated and cross the index finger over the middle finger and draw the fingers forwards and backwards over the lesion.

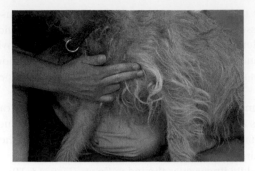

Figure 6.12 *Friction technique*. Place the fingers on the lesion to be treated and place two finger pads working side by side and draw across the lesion forwards and backwards.

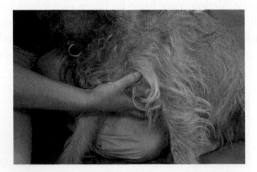

Figure 6.13 *Friction technique*. Place the thumb pad on the lesion to be treated. Flex and extend the distal interphalangeal joint over.

surface, and the amplitude of the movement should be appropriate for the size of the tissue being treated.

Friction massage is used to loosen adhesions and adherent scar tissue by loading and stretching the collagen fibres following an injury or strain. This will maintain and restore the normal mobility of the tissues. In tendons, removing any adhesions between the gliding surfaces of the tendon and its sheath will optimise their function. In ligaments, the prevention and removal of adhesions between the ligament and its neighbouring structures improves their function. In muscle tissue, the breaking down of adhesions allows the muscle fibres to work more freely and maintains their ability to broaden when required. Chemically, the cells irritated or damaged by the friction massage will release a histamine-like substance that will cause vasodilation and cause local circulatory changes.

The use of friction massage in animals must be performed with caution, as in humans the pressure applied during a friction will often cause discomfort or pain and then the patient will describe a numbing effect occurring as you continue. If you were to apply this technique in an animal at this depth, you may lose compliance or cause the animal to become aggressive. Therefore, choose the patients you use this technique on with care or modify the technique that you use if you feel the animal would not tolerate deep pressure.

Trigger point massage or release

Trigger points occur within skeletal muscle and are always associated with a dysfunction but they are not always painful. The definition of a trigger point is *'a hyper-irritable focus within a taut band of skeletal muscle and located in muscular tissue and/or its fascia'.*

Trigger points develop within muscle tissue following a sustained depolarisation of the endplate within the muscle fibre, which causes a prolonged shortening of the sarcomeres. The contraction of the sarcomeres will increase their energy consumption and causes compression on the local capillaries resulting in local hypoxia. The increased energy demands and reduced circulation will cause tissue distress, which in turn causes the release of bradykinins and prostaglandins. These cause pain and along with histamine activate the release of acetylcholine. This is a positive feedback loop and will continue until the trigger point is deactivated.

Trigger points can be active, passive, primary or secondary.

Active trigger points

These will be painful on palpation and are usually associated with existing pain or dysfunction in the animal. The amount of pain experienced with active trigger points is variable and depending on their severity, they can cause a great deal of referred pain. The size of a trigger point does not affect the amount of pain experienced. It is the irritability of the trigger point that influences the amount of pain felt and as the irritability decreases, the trigger point can become passive.

Passive trigger points

These are associated with a restriction of movement and can be found in clinically normal patients. Often these can be described as 'knots' in muscle tissue. They will be less painful on palpation and can be formed where there are weak/fatigued muscles or when tissues are overused or overstretched.

Primary trigger points

These will arise as a result of an injury, following a virus or disease (such as flu that can cause muscle pain and tenderness) and as a result of the abnormal stresses (or muscle overload) placed on myofascial tissue. They will cause pain and muscle guarding of a painful area that increase the muscle stress elsewhere and may then cause secondary trigger points.

Secondary trigger points

These arise from irritation elsewhere such as active trigger points and from visceral disease. It is important to note that trigger points arising from visceral disturbances are unlikely to respond to therapeutic techniques and warrant a referral back to the primary veterinary surgeon for further investigation.

The detection of trigger points within muscle tissue needs careful palpation. Active trigger points will cause a discrete area of tenderness and a taut band but caution is needed not to palpate them too deeply as the muscle they are located within may be in spasm or hypertonic causing the animal to react violently and possibly aggressively. Passive trigger points can be more difficult to palpate as they will not be painful but the taut band will still be identifiable. A muscle can have multiple trigger points within its tissue and often in these cases the pain will be more generalised. To treat many trigger points in one muscle will be very painful and is likely to reduce compliance of the animal. In these cases, the selection of a few trigger points on the initial treatment will be more successful and the rest can be treated in the next session. It is important to treat/eliminate trigger points to not only relieve the pain exhibited by the animal but also to restore function to the muscles and to prevent further problems.

The treatment of trigger points is especially important in sporting or working animals as they need full joint range of movement and a fully functioning myofascial system to perform to the best of their ability. The presence of trigger points in muscle will reduce the flexibility, power and endurance of the muscle that they are found in. Trigger points in the paraspinal muscles especially can cause lameness and/or stiffness. The pain caused by trigger points will also affect the active and passive stretching of a muscle leading to reduced range of movement and if prolonged can cause muscle spasm, which will lead to adaptive shortening of the muscle. The adaptive shortening may continue to present as a problem even when pain has been reduced and this will lead to muscle imbalance. It is very rare to see neurological signs, such as atrophy caused by trigger points; however, it may occur if the spasm does entrap a peripheral nerve. Trigger points are self-sustaining, and lameness or dysfunction can often remain after an original injury has healed due to a secondary trigger point around the affected area and they will remain indefinitely until deactivated or eliminated.

There are a number of treatment methods that can be used to deactivate trigger points. These include manual techniques such as ischaemic compression or stretching, electrical techniques such as electrical nerve or muscle stimulation, electrotherapy such as ultrasound or laser and for trained veterinarians, dry needling (acupuncture) or a combination of all of the above-mentioned techniques.

Ischaemic compression (also known as manual compression, inhibitory pressure or pressure release) is a very commonly used technique for trigger point deactivation. This technique is where a continuous, gentle, vertical pressure is applied to the taut band of muscle until the tension is released. The pressure is usually exerted by a finger or thumb pad, but the heel of hand or elbow can be used depending on the size of the animal. The pressure applied can be slowly increased until the tissue is felt to relax or 'give'. This can be accompanied by a sighing or a lowering of the head. The vertical pressure from ischaemic compression is thought to 'squash' the sarcomeres in the affected area thus lengthening them, that is, like applying a vertical pressure on a balloon will push the air in it horizontally. Once a trigger point has been deactivated, the muscle should always be stretched afterwards (Figure 6.14).

Once trigger points have been deactivated, it is important to educate owners on the prevention of trigger points arising in the future. In sporting animals, avoiding repetitive activities; exercising animals until they are exhausted and running on very hard, soft or uneven ground can cause trigger points. If an animal becomes very cold and or sleeps on inappropriate bedding this can also cause trigger points.

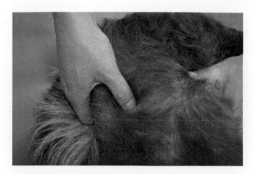

Figure 6.14   *Ischaemic compression.* Place the thumb on the band of taut muscle and press verti-cally down.

Myofascial release

This is a soft-tissue technique where myofascial restrictions are released through sus-tained pressure to improve movement and to reduce pain. Fascial planes stretch throughout the body and symptoms can be exhibited anywhere along the fascial plane. There are many recognised techniques (too many for this text to describe), but they can be categorised broadly as static and dynamic techniques.

The connective tissue or fascia responds to myofascial release techniques because it has viscoelastic properties. All connective tissues contain ground substance, col-lagen, reticulin and elastin, with fascia containing a large proportion of collagen. Collagen (as stated in Chapter 3) resists tensile forces and has a crimped appear-ance. When fascia becomes strained, it tightens leading to reduced flexibility, reduced mobility and pain. Fascial strain can occur as a result of trauma, infection, imbal-ance and restriction or reduced mobility in a joint. Over time the tightened fascia can solidify, shorten, reorganise itself along the line of stress and bind to joints and mus-cle tissue, which will increase the amount of restriction or dysfunction. If the fascia remains restricted and 'bound/tied down', then it can alter the alignment of the joints and further reduce overall function. This occurs because the collagen adapts to the stress by increasing the amount of cross links, dehydration of the ground substance, formation of adhesions and anchoring of the fascia to adjacent structures.

The aim of myofascial release is to increase the water content of the fascia, stretch the elastic component of collagen and to break the adherent cross links. This will restore the flexibility of the fascia allowing normal joint motion and postural align-ment to return. When performing myofascial release or MFR, the therapist has to palpate the fascia to feel for restriction, which will be a dense, thickened or hard feel-ing within the tissue. The therapist's hands take up the stretch within the system and when resistance is felt, a consistent gentle pressure is applied. The pressure should be held for 1–2 minutes or until the fascia is felt to release. The sustained pressure is held to allow plastic deformation of the collagen to occur and is released slowly to allow the tissue to relax back to its original length. The pressure must be released slowly as a sudden release of the fascia could cause a 'rebound' of the tissue, which will negate the effect of treatment. MFR cannot be performed forcibly as the pressure

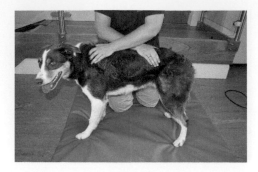

Figure 6.15   *Cross-hand MFR technique.* Cross the hands over one another and direct the pressure away from each hand towards the ends of the muscle being treated until a restriction is reached.

has to be applied gently, because the fascia will meet the forcible movement with equal resistance.

When performing MFR, it is important to note that the amount of force used directly relates to the elasticity of the fibres and the speed of the release relates to the viscosity of the tissue fluid. Therefore, performing MFR slowly and gently will permanently lengthen the fascia. The efficacy of MFR (as with all manual techniques) is dependent on the therapist's ability to assess the tissues and apply the correct amount of force and speed to the tissue to achieve a release.

Some of the most common techniques used for MFR are the cross-hand release, where the hands are crossed over one another and the pressure is directed away from each hand towards the ends of the muscle being treated until a restriction is reached (Figure 6.15). The longitudinal single- or double-handed release is where the hands are placed at the end of the muscle and pressure is directed along the fibre orientation. During the treatment, the therapist's hands must remain in contact with the tissues and the release is continued without interruption. Heat can be applied to the area to be treated before treatment. This will warm the tissues and relax the muscles that can help improve the efficacy of treatment. Following MFR, stretching will reinforce treatment by elongating the muscle and fascia, and restore movement.

Joint movements

Passive movements
These are anatomical movements that would normally be performed by the patient. But, due to muscle inactivity or muscle atrophy, they are performed by an external force without resistance or assistance from the patient. They are used to maintain range of movement, soft-tissue extensibility and thus function of a joint (or leg) when the patient is unable to move the joint due to muscle or nerve injury or disease. The amount of motion will always be within the available range of movement. The person performing a passive movement must be sensitive to the motion and how far to push it (Figure 6.16).

When performing passive movements, the therapist can choose to move single joints, several joints in sequence or several joints simultaneously. The choice of technique will be influenced by the aim of performing a passive movement. They

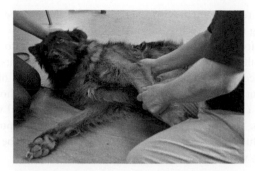

Figure 6.16 *Performing passive elbow extension.* With your dog lying on its side, place one hand behind the elbow and upper part of the leg. Gently bring the lower part of the leg away from the head as if trying to straighten the elbow.

can be used to maintain or increase range of movement, to maintain extensibility of muscles or to re-educate normal movement/function. When treating loss of range of movement, all movements should be addressed in that joint that are restricted with each movement being taken to its limit and held in this position. The muscles that benefit from passive movements are the bi-articulate or multi-articulate muscles (two or more joint muscles). The joints they cross need to be positioned so that a stretch can be achieved throughout the length of the muscle. The re-education of normal movement by using passive movements is especially important after injury to the nervous system by using functional movement patterns (see chapter 7).

When performing passive movements, there are many things to consider:

- Position of the animal – the patients need to be comfortable, relaxed, warm and supported, otherwise they will not allow movement to occur without resistance.
- Position of yourself – you need to be able to reach the joint/s being moved comfortably at the beginning and end of the movement without straining.
- Position of your hands – the joint/s to be moved should be held proximally and distally as close as possible without hindering the movement or allowing excessive movement to occur around the joint/s. The holds will be specific for different movements and if this needs to be changed during the movement, it has to be done smoothly as the animal could become tense.
- How the joint is grasped – for the animal to feel supported, the joint/s need to be grasped firmly but not excessively so as to cause discomfort as this will cause the animal to become more tense' the passive movement will become ineffectives towards the end of range, the skin will become more stretched and the grasp may need to be relaxed slightly to prevent dragging across the skin.
- How you move the joint/s – the movement should be slow, steady, rhythmical and in a functional plane taking care not to put excessive rotation on the joint/s if you are not intentionally moving in that direction.
- Which joints you are treating – when treating many joints, it is important to decide which order you are treating them to achieve slightly different goals. An immobilised patient would benefit from being treated distally to proximally in the affected leg to aid venous return.
- Application of accessory movements – as the motion is performed, a slight traction (or distraction) may be given and a slight compression at the end of range

to encourage more movement. However, these should only be performed when sufficient training in these techniques has been given.

- Assess feedback from the animal – your position needs you to be able to watch the animal carefully throughout a passive movement to assess its response as your technique will need to be modified if the patient shows signs of discomfort. The patient should not be forced if resistance to the movement is shown.

There are some conditions where caution should be observed when performing passive movements. They are hypermobility, non-ossified joints (puppies), total joint replacements and during pregnancy. In all these cases, joints can be moved past their physiological limits, which will cause more harm to the patient.

Accessory movements

These are movements that occur as part of a normal joint movement, but cannot be performed in isolation or voluntarily by the patient. They have a very small range of movement, but are essential for normal joint function in active and passive ROM. Therefore, a loss of an accessory movement will result in a restriction in joint movement. Examples of accessory movements are glides, distraction, compression and rotation.

Side glides: Firmly grasp the joint to be treated on the medial and lateral sides as close as possible to the joint surfaces. The gliding motion is applied as the hands are moved towards each other (Figure 6.17).

Distraction: Firmly grasp the joint distally and proximally and draw the hands apart (Figure 6.18).

Compression: Firmly grasp the joint as in distraction technique and draw the hands together (Figure 6.19).

Rotation: Firmly grasp the joint distally and proximally, stabilise the proximal part of the joint and move the distal hand either medially or laterally to create the rotation (Figure 6.20).

To perform accessory movements, the joint has to be placed in an open-packed position where the joint surfaces are not congruent, and the tension on the capsule, ligaments, muscles and tendons is relaxed. This is midway between the extremes of the active joint movement in opposing directions.

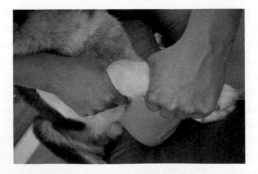

Figure 6.17 *Accessory side glide technique.* Carpal side glide, with the dog sitting flex the carpus and firmly grasp on the medial and lateral sides as close as possible to the joint surfaces. Move the hands towards each other to glide the joint surfaces across each other.

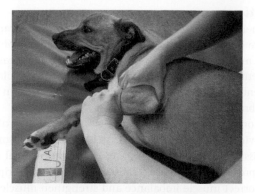

Figure 6.18   *Accessory distraction*. Elbow distraction, firmly grasp the joint distally and proximally and draw the hands apart to gap the joint surfaces.

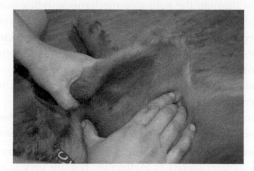

Figure 6.19   *Accessory compression*. Elbow compression, fully flex the joint and firmly grasp distally and proximally, press the hands together to compress the joint surfaces.

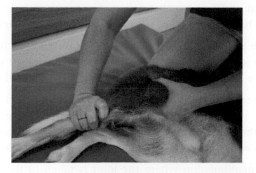

Figure 6.20   *Accessory rotation technique*. Stifle rotation, firmly grasp the joint distally and proximally, stabilise the proximal part of the joint and move the distal hand either medially or laterally to create the rotation.

Joint mobilisations

Different practitioners, chiropractors, osteopaths and physiotherapists use different techniques to move joints. Physiotherapists tend to use joint mobilisations that are passive rhythmical movements or oscillations that are used to treat stiffness or pain. They are also repetitive and localised techniques, which are selected following a thorough assessment of the patient's signs and symptoms and can be applied to the peripheral or vertebral joints.

Joint mobilisations are used to restore normal painless range of movement. This is achieved by relieving pain, reducing muscle spasm, improving soft-tissue pliability, restoring normal tissue-fluid exchange and restoration of normal movement. Once joint mobility is improved through mobilisation, the correct prescription of follow-on exercise will also correct muscle imbalance and strengthen muscles to help stabilise any unstable joints. The mechanical effects of oscillatory movements on a joint include improved cartilage nutrition, intervertebral disc nutrition and metabolism of soft tissue. The neurological effects include stimulation of mechanoreceptors that in turn will reduce pain through the pain gate mechanism, reflex inhibition of muscle contractions and reduced intra-articular pressure around the joint through stimulation of mechanoreceptors and nociceptors. In vertebral mobilisations, stimulation of mechanoreceptors in the facet joint capsules can produce reflex effects on the vertebral and leg musculature. The reflex changes that occur as a result of joint mobilisation can also have an effect, such as smooth muscle tone, pulse rate, cardiac output and blood pressure.

When applying joint mobilisations, the amount of pressure or force used is graded on a scale of I–V based on Maitland's approach to joint movement (Figure 6.21).

Grade I: These are small-amplitude movements in early or comfortable ROM for the patient. They may be considered as ineffective, but are very useful for extremely painful patients where muscle spasm occurs on gentle passive movements. They have a pain-relieving effect on the patient.

Grade II: These are large-amplitude movements in comfortable ROM, but moving more into mid range. They remain in the range where muscle spasm is not provoked and again have a pain-relieving effect and also a vascular effect.

Grade III: These are large-amplitude movements up to the limit of ROM. They are done when pain is felt at end ROM and can cause discomfort to the patient but should not induce muscle spasm. They have a vascular and mobilising effect.

Grade IV: These are small-amplitude movements done at the limit of available ROM with the joint at maximal stretch. They are done when there is very little pain associated with the joint and they do not provoke muscle spasm. They again can cause discomfort whilst being performed and are used to mobilise a stiff joint.

Grade V: This is a manipulation where the joint is taken to the limit of its range and then moved with high velocity through a small amplitude before the patient is aware of the movement occurring. The movement is often accompanied by a click. This movement is most commonly used by chiropractors and should only be performed after comprehensive training.

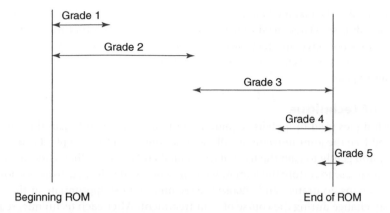

Figure 6.21 *Maitland's scale.* The amount of pressure exerted on a joint for the different grades of passive movement on the Maitland's scale.

The grade and speed of movement used will depend on the irritability of the joint to be treated. Slow gentle rhythm for grade I for severe-pain patients and a staccato technique for patients with minimal symptoms are used. The length of mobilisation is also dependent on the irritability. Generally very painful joints should be mobilised for no longer than 20–30 seconds and this repeated 1–2 times to minimise aggravation of symptoms. The non-irritable joints can be mobilised for a minute at a time and repeated 4–6 times. As a general rule, treatment should always be started gently and the amount of force and duration can be increased after reassessment of your initial treatment techniques. It can sometimes be necessary to do less treatment initially to gain compliance before increasing force or duration in the next treatment session. In some cases, when higher grade mobilisations are being used, it is important to warn the owner that the animal may experience some discomfort immediately post treatment, but this will not last.

Contraindications

The absolute contraindications to joint mobilisations are:
Malignancy of the bone
Compression of the spinal cord on imaging
Central nervous system disease
Acute dislocations
Active inflammatory and infective arthritis
Bone disease
Unstable fractures
Vascular disease
Aggressive or highly fearful dog
Owner lack of understanding or anxiety

Care needs to be taken when the patient is pregnant, hypermobile or had previous metastatic disease. (They need to have radiographic evidence that the joint you are treating does not have any metastases.) If a joint is painful as a result of increased mobility (hypermobility), then to passively mobilise the joint can be harmful and cause more pain.

Types of technique

The techniques used to mobilise a joint are primarily designed to gap the joint surfaces and free the joint movement. All mobilisations need to be applied confidently, skilfully and gently to gain the trust of the animal and owner. When choosing which technique to use to restore the joint movement, you need to be able to assess how the joint is moving accurately and choose the technique most appropriate at that time. This may change during the course of your treatment. After each technique, reassess how the joint is moving and use the most effective technique last. There is no one treatment that can cure all abnormalities of joint movement and equally you may find yourself using different techniques on different joints, especially in spinal cases. Each joint problem presentation will be unique to that individual and the selection of the techniques needs to be done carefully and to be adapted if required.

When assessing the joint for movement, place the joint into the midpoint of its available range and palpate for tenderness, spasm, thickening around the joint and reduced accessory movement. It may also be necessary to place an overpressure on the joint (where the joint is gently forced past its end of range) to determine the end feel of the joint and observe how the symptoms react. Some examples of markers for assessment could be: ROM (active and passive), neurological signs, lameness, degree of pain on palpation and changes in muscle spasm. These markers can be used between techniques, but are also important between treatment sessions to assess the effectiveness of treatment. The assessment of a joint movement and pain cannot be learnt from a book, neither can the ability to develop, adapt and modify techniques. These are based on experience and it can take years to develop your feel.

There are numerous vertebral mobilisations that can be used and some are localised (specific to one vertebral segment) or regional techniques (treating numerous segments). The techniques vary slightly depending on which region you are treating in the spine and mobilisations can be done with the spine in neutral, side flexion, rotation, flexion or extension depending on the desired effect. The techniques described are simple mobilisations. It is recommended that further training is completed to learn the more specific mobilisations.

Dorsal–ventral pressures

These are useful in the thoracic and lumbar spine and can be done directly or indirectly on the spinous processes to assess the vertebral segment or unilaterally to assess one facet joint specifically. Direct D–V is where the thumb or ulnar border of the hand is placed onto the spinous process and pressure is applied directly downwards (Figure 6.22). An indirect D–V is where the thumb and index knuckle or two knuckles are pressed downwards on the transverse processes simultaneously (Figure 6.23). A painful response would be a muscle twitch of the paraspinal muscles or the animal moving away from the pressure. A unilateral D–V is where thumb pressure is applied directly on one transverse process. This will produce a rotational movement around

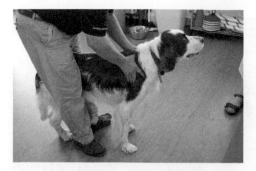

Figure 6.22 *Direct dorsoventral pressure.* With the animal in sitting, standing or sternal lying position, place the thumb or ulnar border of the hand onto the spinous process and apply pressure directly down.

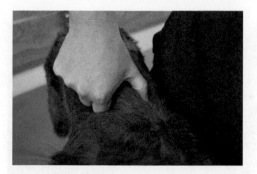

Figure 6.23 *Bilateral dorsoventral pressure.* With the animal in sitting, standing or sternal lying position, place the thumb and index knuckle onto the transverse processes at the same level, and pressure is directed downwards simultaneously.

that vertebral segment (Figure 6.24). Again a painful response will produce a muscle twitch or movement from the animal. The end feel of the movement can also be assessed.

Transverse pressures or side glides
These can be done locally or regionally with the dog in standing or lying position. It is easiest to use the local technique when the animal is in lateral recumbency. Using the thumb, locate the spinous process of the level you wish to treat and push it towards the floor (Figure 6.25). The regional technique is where the hands grasp the spine at the level you wish to treat and push the spine away whilst the other hand pulls the hips or shoulders in the opposite direction (Figure 6.26).

Rotations
These can be done effectively in the lumbar spine. With the animal in lateral recumbency, stabilise the lower side of the spinous process to be treated. Then use the pelvis to rotate the lumbar spine by rolling it backwards (Figure 6.27).

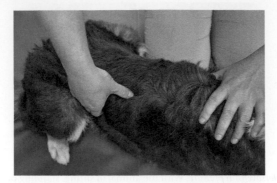

Figure 6.24   *Unilateral dorsoventral pressure.* With the animal in sitting, standing or sternal lying position, place thumb on one transverse process and direct the pressure downwards.

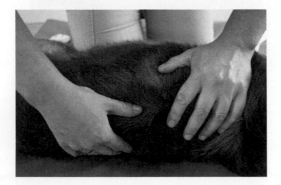

Figure 6.25   *Specific side bends.* Place the animal in lateral recumbency. Use the thumb locate the spinous process of the level you wish to treat and push it towards the floor.

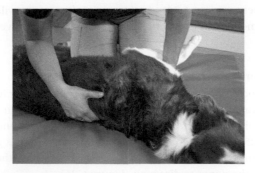

Figure 6.26   *Regional side bends.* Place the animal in lateral recumbency. Grasp the spine at the level you wish to treat and push the spine away whilst the other hand draws the shoulders up in the opposite direction.

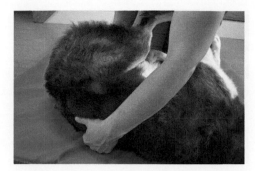

Figure 6.27 *Lumbar rotation*. Place the animal in lateral recumbency. Stabilise the lower side of the spinous process you wish to treat, use the pelvis to rotate the lumbar spine by rolling it backwards.

Traction

This is a technique where a sustained or rhythmically intermittent force is applied along the longitudinal axis of the body part. The angle of force can be subtly changed to provide a dorsal, ventral or lateral pull on the joint. Traction can also be graded by Maitland's scale as described earlier. Traction is used to mobilise stiff joints, reduce muscle spasm, relieve pain, stretch muscle and connective tissue and improve circulation. It is also thought that traction can help reduce neurological symptoms by having a 'suction' effect on herniated disc material.

Intermittent traction can improve circulation, which will reduce swelling of surrounding tissues and epidural space and improve the tissue-fluid exchange. The movement will stimulate mechanoreceptors of the joint capsules modifying abnormal joint movement patterns and inhibit nociceptor activity giving pain relief. Traction can also relieve the inflammatory reaction of nerve roots and can contribute to resorption and regression of the herniated disc material and create an alternating stretching and relaxation of adjacent soft-tissue structures.

In animals, traction is applied manually, and hence a great amount of your success will rely on technique. The technique for vertebral traction depends on the area of the spine you are treating and the size of animal to be treated. In smaller animals, traction can be applied by one person (Figure 6.28) or two people (Figure 6.29), but in larger dogs, it may be more appropriate to use two people for traction. The cranial hand or person stabilises the animal and the caudal hand provides the traction force.

Contraindications for traction

Infection
Neoplasm
Bilateral pars inter-articular defect
Grade 2 or higher spondylolisthesis
Fractures
Presence of metal work within the spine

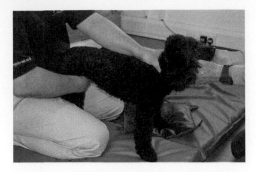

Figure 6.28 *One-person thoracic traction.* With the animal in standing, sitting or sternal lying position, place one hand on the cervical spine and the other hand around the pelvis. The cranial hand stabilises the animal and the caudal hand provides the traction force.

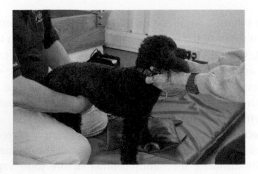

Figure 6.29 *Two-people thoracic traction.* One person stabilises the animal at the cervical spine and the other person holds the pelvis. The caudal person draws the pelvis away to provide the traction force.

When selecting which manual therapies to use, the body must always be thought of as a balance between all the movement systems. Restriction in the joint movement will cause restriction in the myofascial system, and pain or imbalance in the nervous system will provoke a response from the muscular system. As physiotherapists, we often have to address many facets of a problem until we get a good response or resolution and the analogy of peeling an onion with many layers is often true.

CHAPTER 7

Common neurological conditions and their rehabilitation

This chapter will describe how to differentiate between an upper motor lesion and a lower motor lesion and how to localise the lesion using clinical examination. Suggested protocols for common neurological cases are suggested, but the reader is reminded that each case is different and regular reviews of the treatment plan are required. Conditions of the brain and cranial nerves will not be covered.

Neurological examination

The neurological examination should follow on from the clinical examination (Chapter 4) where a neurological condition is suspected. It is important that a full clinical examination is conducted first so that potential mistakes are avoided. A classic example of this is the sudden onset non-weight bearing in both back legs in a Rottweiler or Labrador Retriever that has ruptured both cranial cruciate ligaments. During the clinical examination, attention should be paid to gait, posture and head carriage.

Lower motor lesion versus upper motor lesion
Lower motor neuron (LMN)
The lower motor neuron cell body lies within the ventral horn. Its axon leaves the ventral nerve root and runs as a peripheral nerve. It then synapses with a muscle. The lower motor neuron is the last nerve in a chain of transmission that results in the contraction of a muscle.

The spinal cord is arranged in segments. Each spinal segment innervates specific muscles. By using a series of neurological reflexes, it is possible to localise the site of a lesion (Figure 7.1).
Signs of LMN damage are:
Reduced or absent muscle tone.

Flaccid paresis or paralysis.

Reduced or absent reflexes.

Early and marked muscle atrophy.

Practical Physiotherapy for Small Animal Practice, First Edition.
Edited by David Prydie and Isobel Hewitt.
© 2015 John Wiley & Sons, Ltd. Published 2015 by John Wiley & Sons, Ltd.
Companion Website: www.wiley.com/go/practical-physiotherapy-for-small-animals

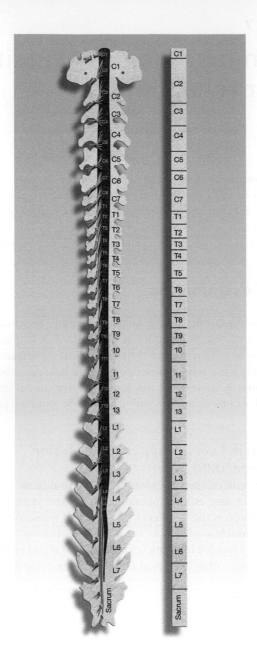

Figure 7.1 *Spinal cord segments*. There are 8 cervical segments, 13 thoracic, 7 lumbar and 3 sacral in dogs and cats. The paired nerve roots leave the spinal cord at their corresponding vertebral foramen. The spinal cord ends at the level of L6–L7.

Table 7.1   UMN or LMN localisation.

Site of lesion	Front legs	Back legs
C1–C5	UMN	UMN
C6–T2	LMN	UMN
T2–L3	Normal	UMN
L4–S3	Normal	LMN
Polyradiculopathy/polyneuropathy	LMN	LMN

Upper motor neuron (UMN)

The upper motor neuron runs from the brain down the spinal cord to eventually synapse with the lower motor neuron. It may consist of more than one nerve, involving, interneurons. The UMN is responsible for initiating a muscle contraction and maintaining correct muscle tone. UMNs also have an inhibitory effect on muscle reflexes.

Signs of UMN damage are:

Normal or increased extensor muscle tone.

Spastic paresis or paralysis.

Normal or increased reflex activity.

Chronic cases will show disuse muscle atrophy (Table 7.1).

Reflexes

Reflexes that test the LMN

Front leg

Withdrawal Reflex (Flexors C6–T2)

With the dog in lateral recumbency, pinch between the toes or nail bed using fingers or artery forceps. This noxious stimulus causes contraction withdrawal of the leg (Figure 7.2).

This is a local or segmental reflex involving individual segments of the spinal cord. It does not depend on the animal feeling the sensation of 'pain'.

Extensor carpi radialis reflex (C7–T2)

With the patient in lateral recumbency, slightly flex the carpus. Tap the area indicated in the picture with a reflex hammer. An intact segment produces a slight extension of the carpus (Figure 7.3).

Biceps brachii reflex – musculocutaneous nerve (C6–C8)

Again with the dog in lateral recumbency, extend the elbow. Place a finger over the insertion of the biceps brachii muscle. Gently tap the finger. The elbow should slightly flex. Note this reflex is less reliable than the two reflexes above and it may not be possible to elicit a reaction even in a normal animal (Figure 7.4).

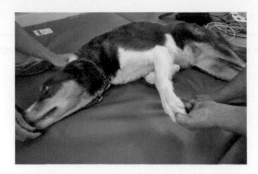

Figure 7.2 *Withdrawal (flexor) Reflex, front leg.* With the dog on its side, pinch between the toes or on the nail bed using finger and thumb or artery forceps. Look for flexion (withdrawal) of the leg.

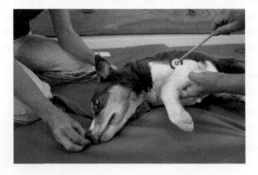

Figure 7.3 *Extensor carpi radialis reflex.* Using a reflex hammer, tap in the proximal ante brachium with carpus slightly flexed. The carpus should slightly extend.

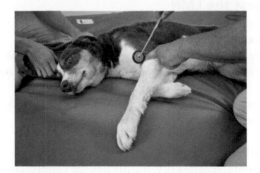

Figure 7.4 *Biceps brachii reflex.* Place a finger over the insertion of the biceps and extend the elbow. Tap the finger with a reflex hammer. The elbow should slightly flex.

Triceps reflex – radial nerve (C7–T1)

Flex the elbow. Using a reflex hammer, tap the triceps tendon close to its insertion onto olecranon. A positive test should result in slight extension of the elbow. Again, this is a less-reliable reflex than the withdrawal and extensor carpi radialis (Figure 7.5).

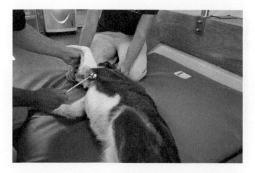

Figure 7.5 *Triceps reflex.* Flex the elbow and gently tap the triceps tendon with a reflex hammer. The elbow should slightly extend.

Back leg
Withdrawal reflex (L4–S2)
With the dog in lateral recumbency and with the hock extended, pinch between the toes or nail bed. The leg should be withdrawn. Try to look for flexion of each individual joint, hip, stifle and hock (Figure 7.6).

Patella reflex – femoral nerve (L4–L6)
With the animal in lateral recumbency, slightly flex and support the stifle. Tap the patella tendon with a reflex hammer. The stifle should extend (Figure 7.7).

Cranial tibial reflex (L6–S1)
Again with the patient in lateral recumbency, support the stifle. Tap the proximal part of the cranial tibial muscle with a reflex hammer. A positive reflex results in flexion of the hock. This reflex is less consistent than the withdrawal and patella reflexes (Figure 7.8).

Gastrocnemius reflex (L7–S1)
Place the patient in lateral recumbency. Cover the distal part of the gastrocnemius muscle with a finger. Strike the finger with a reflex hammer. Hock extension should

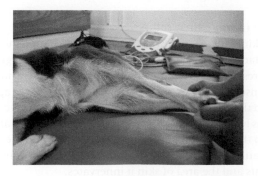

Figure 7.6 *Withdrawal reflex, back leg.* Slightly extend the hock. Pinch between the toes and watch for flexion of each joint.

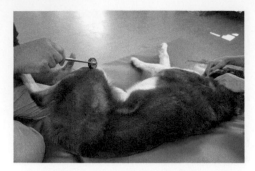

Figure 7.7 *Patella reflex.* Flex and support the stifle. Gently tap the patella tendon. The stifle should extend.

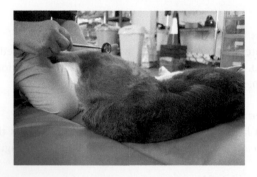

Figure 7.8 *Cranial tibial reflex.* Support the stifle and gently tap the proximal part of the cranial tibial muscle. Look for hock flexion.

be observed. Again, this reflex is not as reliable as the withdrawal and patella reflexes (Figure 7.9).

Other reflexes

Perineal reflex (S1–Cd5)

Gently pinch the perineum with artery forceps. Look for contraction of the anal sphincter and tail flexion (Figure 7.10).

Cutaneous trunci (panniculus) reflex

Gently pinch the skin with artery forceps on either side of midline at various points from T2–L5. An intact reflex will result in a twitch of the skin (Figure 7.11).

This reflex is present in the thoracolumbar area, but absent in the cervical and sacral areas. The sensory nerves of this reflex enter the spinal cord approximately two vertebrae cranial to the area being tested. The efferent nerves leave the spinal cord at C8–T1. With lesions between T3–L3, there is a cut-off of the reflex approximately two vertebrae caudal to the location of the lesion. Cranial to lesion the reflex is normal.

Skin sensation can also be used to localise a lesion. Table 7.2 lists each nerve, its spinal cord segments and the area of skin it innervates.

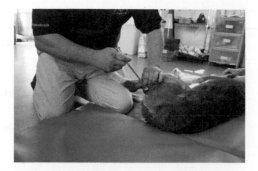

Figure 7.9 *Gastrocnemius reflex.* Place a finger over the distal gastrocnemius and tap the finger. Look for hock extension.

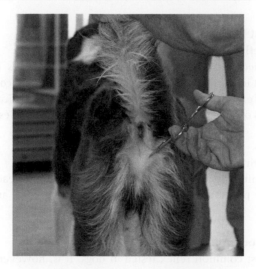

Figure 7.10 *Perineal reflex.* Gently pinch the skin on the perineum. Look for contraction of the anal sphincter and flexion of the tail.

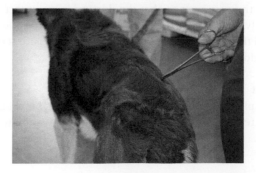

Figure 7.11 *Cutaneous trunci (panniculus) reflex.* Start by gently pinching the skin either side over the wings of the ilium. The skin should twitch over the area stimulated. If a twitch is absent, the test is repeated moving cranially on both sides until a positive result is elicited.

Table 7.2 Neural segments of each nerve and the area of skin innervated.

Nerve	Spinal cord segment	Area of skin innervated
Musculocutaneous	C6–C8	Medial ante brachium
Radial	C7–T2	Cranial aspect of ante brachium and foot except the fifth digit
Median and ulna	C8–T2	Caudal aspect of ante brachium and the fifth digit
Femoral	L3–L6	Medial aspect of back leg and first digit
Sciatic	L6–S2	Craniolateral and caudal aspect of the back leg distal to the stifle

Reflexes that test both UMN and LMN
Cross-extensor reflex
This reflex is carried out when doing the withdrawal reflexes (Figures 7.2 and 7.6). While the test leg is observed for withdrawal (flexion), the contra-lateral leg is observed for sign of extension. If this is seen in the front legs, it indicates a UMN lesion cranial to C6. If it is observed in the back legs, it indicates a UMN lesion cranial to L4.

Postural reflexes.
These reflexes require an intact nervous system.

They test the animal's spacial awareness, the relationship of each leg to its environment and body position. They also affect muscle tone, joint angles and weight bearing.

Conscious proprioception
This test is the most common reflex tested in dogs. It is, however, difficult to perform in cats. The hopping reflex (Figure 7.14) is the preferred postural reflex in cats (Figure 7.12).

With the animal standing squarely on all four legs, support the dog to take most of its weight. Turn the paw over so that the dorsum is in contact with the ground. Observe how quickly the dog replaces the foot to the normal position. The test should be repeated several times. Conscious proprioception deficits are seen in a number of neurological conditions.

Sliding paper test
A piece of paper is placed under the weight-bearing foot. The paper is slowly pulled laterally. A normal response is for the dog to pick the foot up and replace it under the body (Figure 7.13).

Hopping reflex
This is the most reliable postural reflex in cats. The patient is held so that most of the weight is on one leg. The patient is then moved laterally. The normal response is to hop on the leg to place it under the body. This reflex is difficult to perform in large breed dogs (Figure 7.14).

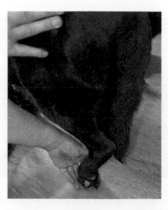

Figure 7.12 *Conscious proprioception.* Support the dog's weight. Gently turn the foot so that the dorsum of the paw is in contact with the ground. Note how long it takes for the dog to replace the foot in the correct position. Repeat several times and on all four legs.

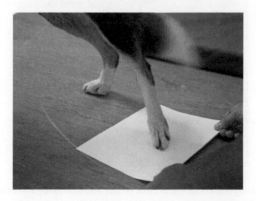

Figure 7.13 *Sliding paper test.* Place a piece of paper under the weight-bearing leg. Gently pull the paper laterally. The dog should lift the leg and replace it under the body.

Visual/tactile placing reflex

These are more complex reflexes and should be additional tests to those above if required. With the visual reflex, the animal is slowly lowered towards a table. The normal response is to reach out for the table before the paw touches (Figures 7.15 and 7.16).

The tactile placing reflex involves covering the animal's eyes. The patient is then lifted and distal part of the thoracic leg is brought towards the edge of a table. The normal response is to reach out and place the foot on the table when the dorsum of the paw comes into contact with the table edge.

Wheelbarrow test

This test can detect subtle thoracic leg ataxia and weakness. The back legs are lifted off the ground by supporting the animal under the abdomen. The animal is then forced to walk forward (Figure 7.17).

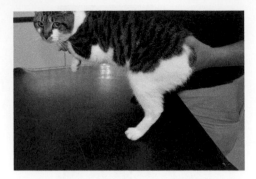

Figure 7.14 *Hopping reflex.* Take the weight off three of the animal's legs so that the remaining leg is taking weight. Gently push the animal laterally. The animal should hop to bring the leg under the body.

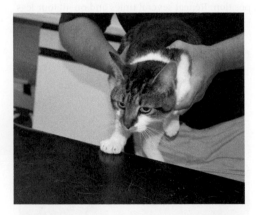

Figure 7.15 *Visual placing reflex.* Lift the animal in the air. Gradually lower towards a table. The normal response is to reach out towards the table before contact is made.

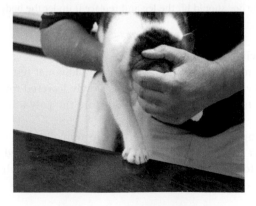

Figure 7.16 *Tactile placing reflex.* With the patient's eyes covered, gently move the distal part of one front leg towards the table edge. The normal response is to reach out for the table when the dorsum of the paw comes in contact with the table edge.

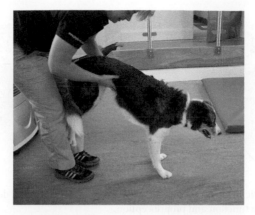

Figure 7.17 *Wheelbarrow test*. Lift the back legs off the ground by supporting the animal under the abdomen. Gently push the animal forward. Normal response is to walk forward on the two front legs.

Hemi-walking

The front and back legs on one side are lifted. The animal is then pushed laterally on the weight-bearing side. This again is a more complex reflex that tests coordination and movement (Figure 7.18).

Pain

Pain must be distinguished from the withdrawal reflex. The sensation of pain is demonstrated by an animal turning its head, vocalising or trying to bite and NOT the withdrawal of the leg.

In a neurological examination, pain is divided into superficial and deep pain. Deep pain is a very good prognostic indicator in spinal cord injury. Superficial pain can be tested by pinching the skin between the toes and observing one of the responses mentioned above. Only in a non-responsive animal should deep pain be assessed. To check for deep pain, use artery forceps to crush a toe or the calcaneous. Absence of a reaction to a deep pain stimulus carries a poor prognosis.

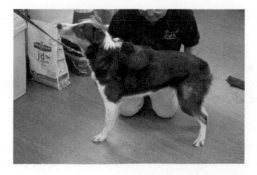

Figure 7.18 *Hemi-walking*. Lift a front and back leg on the same side. Gently push the animal laterally. Normal response is to hop with both the weight-bearing legs.

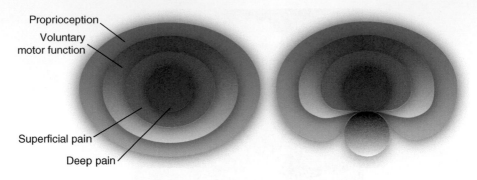

Figure 7.19   Schematic representation of spinal cord showing the depth of deep pain, superficial pain, voluntary motor function and proprioception.

Reflexes are lost (and recovered) in a set order. An animal will lose proprioception first, followed by voluntary motor function, superficial pain and finally deep pain (Figure 7.19). One of the authors (DP) is amazed and disturbed by the overzealousness of veterinarians for testing for deep pain. If an animal can walk, there is no point in testing for deep pain. It will only subject the animal to unnecessary suffering.

Rehabilitation techniques

A variety of techniques are used to try to return the neuromuscular system to normality. The practicality of these techniques will be discussed rather than the theory.

Muscle tone
In spinal cord injury, the legs often have increased (spastic) or decreased (flaccid) muscle tone.

Techniques to reduce muscle tone in hypertonic (spastic) muscles
Slow stroking
The affected muscles and surrounding area are gently stroked. This has the effect of relaxing the muscle spindles and decreasing tension in muscle fibres.

Rhythmical massage
Deep-tissue massage (Chapter 6) is performed in a rhythmical manner paying particular attention to the insertion of the muscle.

Prolonged icing
The affected muscles have ice packs or ice cubes applied directly to the muscle belly for 5–10 minutes. This decreases nerve conduction velocity and hence decreases spindle firing.

Rhythmical rocking

The body and proximal legs are passively rocked for 5–10 minutes. Care must be taken when and where the animal is touched as pressure will stimulate muscle contraction.

Deep tendon pressure

This can be done manually by digital pressure applied to tendons. It is also possible to use the animal's own body weight to stretch the tendons. Make the animal stand squarely on its legs. Gently apply downward pressure and release in a bouncing manner.

Slow PROM

Extensor spasticity can also be broken by flexing the joints in the leg. Start with the toes and flex. Keeping the toes flexed, now flex the carpus/hock, then the elbow/stifle and then the shoulder/hip. Hold the leg in flexion and then gently extend and flex the leg by a very small amount. Do this is in a rhythmical manner. The withdrawal reflex can also be used to encourage reflex movement that in itself will help reduce spasticity.

Techniques to increase muscle tone in hypotonic (flaccid) muscles

Tapping

The affected muscle group is tapped with the fingertips repeatedly to encourage muscle contraction. This can be done in lying or standing position. This can also be used to improve the timing of the muscle contraction (Figure 7.20).

Brushing

The affected muscle group is brushed rapidly with a soft hairbrush to stimulate a contraction (Figure 7.21a).

Vibration

A vibrator or vibration of the hands applied directly to the muscle belly can stimulate muscle contraction. It is best used after brushing and with the muscle in stretch (Figure 7.21b).

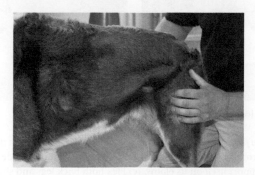

Figure 7.20 *Tapping.* The flaccid muscle group repeatedly with the fingertips to stimulate the muscle to contract.

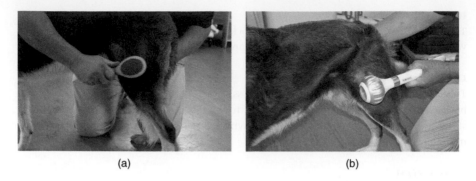

(a)   (b)

Figure 7.21   (a) *Brushing*. A soft hairbrush is used to rapidly brush over the affected muscle belly. (b) A vibrator being used to stimulate muscle contraction.

Quick ice
An ice pack is applied to the muscle belly for a maximum of 15 seconds. Alternatively, an ice cube can be applied to palmer/planter surface of the paw for up to 15 seconds.

Joint compressions (Chapter 6)
These should be performed three repetitions five times daily to stimulate the joint proprioceptors.

Other neurological rehabilitation techniques
Transitions
These are important part of recovery in the spinal patient. Many neurological patients will have to relearn how to go from lateral recumbency to sternal recumbency (Figure 7.22), sternal recumbency to sitting (Figure 7.23), from sitting to

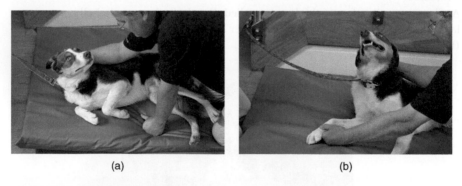

(a)   (b)

Figure 7.22   *Transition from lateral recumbency to sternal recumbency.* (a) With dog lying on its side, guide its head up to promote body movement. (b) Move the front downside leg under the body so that the dog can support itself on its elbow. (c) Flex both back legs and shift the weight of the back of the dog to be centred between the back legs. (d) Flex the upper front leg and position the elbow under the dog. Do the sequence in reverse. Three repetitions five times daily. (e) Also transition to sphinx lying by shifting the position of the downside back leg and adjusting the rear weight evenly.

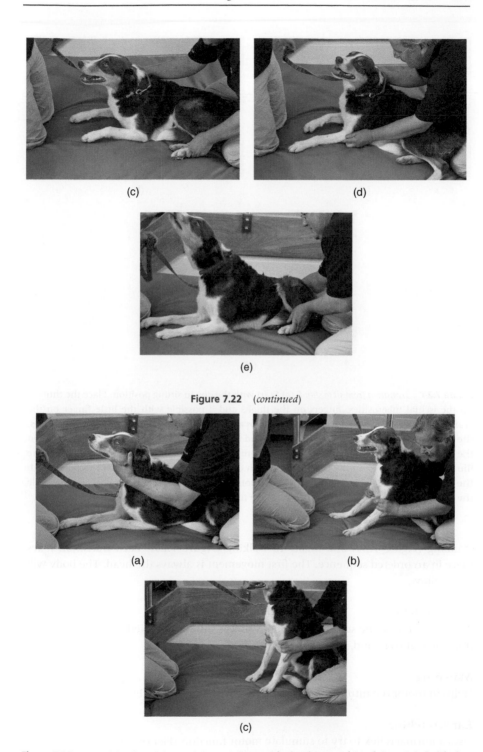

(c)

(d)

(e)

Figure 7.22   (*continued*)

(a)

(b)

(c)

Figure 7.23   *Transition from lying to sitting.* (a) Start with the dog in sphinx lying. Gently lift the head taking care not to hyperextend the neck. (b) and (c) Walk the dog's front legs backwards. Chest support may be required. Return to the sphinx lying position by slowly walking the front legs forward. If extensor spasticity is present, press gently on the cranial aspect of the elbow with the thumbs. Three repetitions five times daily.

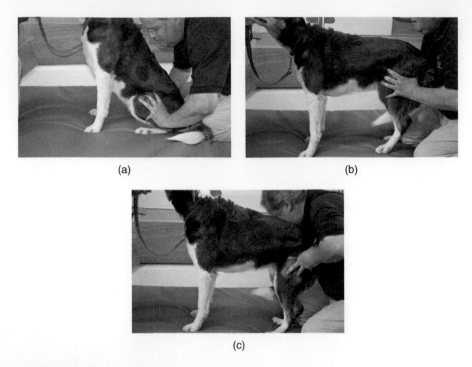

(a)   (b)

(c)

Figure 7.24 *Transition from sit to stand.* (a) Start with the dog in sitting position. Place the thumbs on the ischial tuberosities, fingers on the thighs and if possible with the little finger on the cranial stifle. (b) Push upwards with the thumbs and caudally with the fingers. For larger dogs, the shoulders can be used to push their rear end upwards while using the fingers to straighten the stifles. (c) To return to the sit position, place the thumbs on the dorsal surface of wings of the ilium and little fingers on the caudal stifle. Push downwards with the hand and forwards with the little fingers. Again with large dogs, the shoulders can be used to push downwards while the hands bend the stifle. Three repetitions five times daily.

standing (Figure 7.24) and finally to walking (Figure 7.25). Each transition takes place in an ordered sequence. The first movement is always the head. The body will then follow.

Foot scratching
Aims to stimulate the sensory neurons. Surfaces should be varied from carpet, flooring, grass, gravel, sand, and so on (Figure 7.26).

Marching
Helps in motor recruitment and can guide motor sequencing (Figure 7.27).

Ear scratching
Uses a normal reflex to try to stimulate motor function (Figure 7.28).

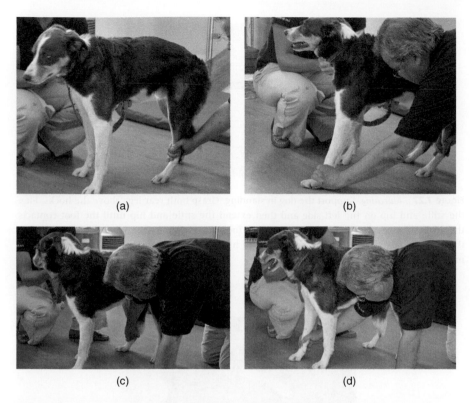

(a) (b)

(c) (d)

Figure 7.25 *Retraining a dog to walk again.* (a) With the dog standing squarely, support the body. Advance the left back leg under the dog. (b) Now advance the left front leg. (c) Followed by the right back leg. (d) And finally the right front leg. Press down on each leg as it contacts the ground. Repeat for six strides. Repeat five times daily.

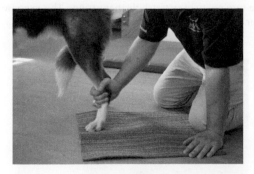

Figure 7.26 *Foot scratching.* With the dog in standing position, place the fingers on the dorsal surface of the paw and thumb just proximal to the main pad. Press down with the fingers while dragging the foot caudally. In the front feet, this can be used to mimic digging and in the back feet to mimic scratching after toileting.

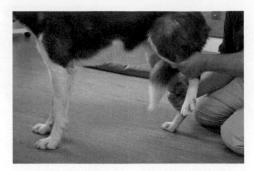

Figure 7.27 *Marching.* Support the dog in standing. Grasp both rear legs above the hocks. Flex the stifle and hip on the left side and then extend the stifle and hip until the foot contacts the ground. Exert downward pressure on the foot. At the same time, as the left leg touches the ground, flex the right leg at the stifle and hip. Continue as for the left leg to produce a marching pattern.

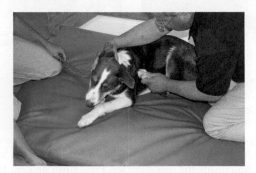

Figure 7.28 *Ear scratching.* Start with the dog sternal recumbency. Bring the dog's head sideways towards the rear legs. At the same time, bring the back leg on the same side towards the ear and mimic scratching. Take care not to overstretch the hamstrings. This exercise can be repeated for scratching the shoulder, chin, face and so on.

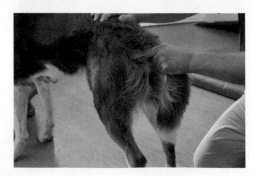

Figure 7.29 *Tail pulls.* Gently grasp the tail head. Gently pull caudally taking care not to lift the tail. The pressure exerted should be the same as pulling a Christmas cracker but not quite to cracking it.

Tail pulls

The dura in the dog continues for some way down the tail. By pulling gently on the tail, the dura further up the spine can be stimulated (Figure 7.29).

Proprioception can be relearnt. Some of the exercises mentioned above stimulate the sensory pathways. More exercises that promote proprioception are covered in Chapter 8.

Neurology rehabilitation protocols

As stated elsewhere in this textbook, these are guideline protocols. Each case will vary and frequent reassessments and replanning are required. Many neurological patients will be unable to stand. Therefore, appropriate bedding and turning is essential to avoid decubit ulcers. For patients with neurogenic bladders and loss of bowl control, appropriate management will be required.

Atlanto-axial subluxation

Most cases are the congenital form of the condition seen in toy breeds such as Pugs and Pomeranians. Dogs are usually under 2 years of age (Figure 7.30).

Signalment. These cases may present acutely or signs may wax and wain. Neck pain is usually present. Other clinical signs can include ataxia, tetraparesis, conscious proprioceptive deficits and increased muscle tone in the front or all four legs. Severe cases will have tetraplegia and respiratory difficulties. Death is a not an uncommon outcome.

Treatment. Surgical cases are usually treated by placing two screws through the articulation between the atlas and axis. Most are placed in a neck cast or brace for several weeks post operatively. With conservative management, the dog is placed in a neck brace for several months.

Rehabilitation. Recovery in a lot of these cases will take several months. Severe cases may not recover at all.

Days 1–14

Focus for management. Preventing further damage. Bladder and bowel management. Surgical cases wound management days 1–10.

Pain relief. NSAIDS +/− opiates as required.

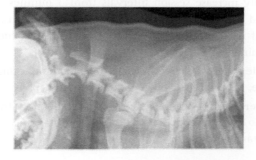

Figure 7.30   Lateral X-ray of a young Pug neck showing atlanto-axial subluxation.

Diet. Most of these cases will be young growing dogs, hence a suitable puppy food as required.

Exercise. These dogs should be on strict cage rest only being taken out for toilet breaks.

Modalities. PEMFT set for pain relief (see manufacturers' instructions).

Manual therapies. Massage legs, especially back legs. Hyper or hypotonic techniques depending on muscle tone. Repeated three times twice daily initially.

Therapeutic exercise. Perform passive ROM of all the legs five repetitions twice daily. Correct positioning of legs into sitting and lying to promote normal tone.

Days 15–30

Focus for management. Continued protection of the area. Bladder and bowel management if required. Management of neck cast or brace. Normalisation of muscle tone and posture.

Pain relief. NSAIDS.

Exercise. Continued cage rest with toilet breaks. No games and no playing with other dogs. No stairs.

Modalities. Continue PEMFT twice weekly.

Manual therapies. Massage all legs. Hyper or hypotonic techniques depending on muscle tone. Repeated three times, five times daily.

Therapeutic exercises. Assisted standing. Transitions, Tapping, Scrunchies to Paws, Wobble Cushion, Wobble Board (see Chapter 8). Start with five repetitions of exercises twice daily and increase as able.

Day 31–90

Focus for management. Increase mobility. Active range of motion. Increase normal movement through the use of transitions. Proprioceptive retraining. Early strengthening.

Pain relief. NSAIDS as required.

Exercise. 5–10 minutes twice daily supported by slings/harness initially if required. No games or playing with other dogs. No stairs.

Modalities. PEMFT at twice-weekly intervals. Introduce hydrotherapy twice weekly. UWTM fill to above elbows. Go at a slow speed to encourage active ROM. Gradually increase session intervals from 3 minutes. If in pool, carry out flexion and extension, and weight-shifting exercises on platforms. Again, gradually build up length of time in the water and introduce short spells of assisted swimming.

Manual therapies. Massage all legs. Hyper or hypotonic techniques depending on muscle tone, as required. Five repetitions five times daily.

Therapeutic exercises. As per above but increase repetitions by 50%. Add Sit to Stand. Down to Sit. Front and Back Leg Lifts, Parastanding with 1 or 2 Books (Chapter 8). Start with five repetitions of exercises twice daily and increase as able.

Days 90–150

> **Focus for management.** Removal of neck brace. Increase activity levels. Strengthening.
>
> **Pain relief.** NSAIDS as required.
>
> **Exercise.** 15 minutes walk twice daily. Start hill work. No playing with other dogs.
>
> **Modalities.** Hydrotherapy weekly. UWTM increase speed and duration. Increase speed. If in the pool, introduce free swimming and gradually increase to 10 minutes.
>
> **Therapeutic exercise.** Continue exercises as for days 31–90, Begin Cavaletti Poles. Figure of Eight, Standing on Swiss Ball (Chapter 8). Repetitions 10 times twice daily.

Cervical disc disease

This protocol is for moderate cases. Severe cases will take much longer time to recover (Figure 7.31).

This condition can occur in almost any breed although Dachshunds, Shih Tzu, Pekingese, Beagles and Cocker Spaniels present most commonly.

Signalment. The age of onset can be young (from 18 months) but peak incidence is usually 3–7 years. They show signs of neck pain that can be severe showing as spasm and rigidity in cervical musculature, can stand with head held down back arched and weight on the back legs, may show tetraparesis, ataxia, proprioceptive deficits, postural reaction deficits or tetraplegia. Dogs may present with UMN lesion to both front and back legs or with LMN lesion to the front legs and UMN lesion to the back legs depending on the location of the disc prolapse.

Diagnosis. X-ray, myelogram, CT or MRI.

Treatment. Conservative management in cases with mild symptoms or owners who are not looking for surgical management.

Surgical Cases Ventral slot to remove disc material and adjacent disc spaces fenestrated.

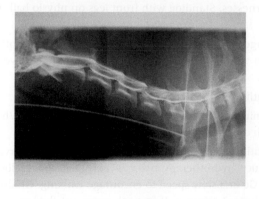

Figure 7.31 Lateral X-ray of a myelogram of a dog showing cervical disc protrusion.

Days 1–14

   Focus for management. Wound management, post-operative swelling. Pain control. Bladder and bowel management.

   Pain Relief. NSAIDS and opiates as required.

   Exercise. Strict cage rest with toilet breaks and organised controlled physiotherapy sessions only.

   Diet. Advise weight loss if required.

   Manual therapies. Massage (Chapter 6) legs, especially back legs. Vibration and tapping or icing and or flexion of legs to treat hypo or hypertonic muscles.

   Modalities. Icing operative site. Twice daily 10 minutes for first 5 days (for post surgery). Laser 3 j/cm^2 at spinal cord. PEMFT set for pain relief (see manufacturers' settings).

   Therapeutic exercise. Perform passive ROM of all joint, all legs, five repetitions twice daily (Chapter 8). Correct positioning of legs into sitting, lying to promote normal tone.

Days 15–30

   Focus for management. Start gentle movement of neck. Increasing ROM of legs. Begin mobilisation.

   Pain relief. NSAIDS.

   Exercise. Build up to 5 minutes twice daily in a harness on level ground.

   Modalities. Laser 3 j/cm^2 at spinal cord. PEMFT set for pain relief (see manufacturers' settings).

   Manual therapies. Gentle traction of spine (Chapter 6).

   Therapeutic exercise. Assisted standing and sit to stand using peanut/slings/hoist/ chest harness to support abdomen (Chapter 9). 2 minutes five times daily or as tolerated by the animal. Active leg withdrawal by tickling feet or gently pinching feet. Slow controlled active head/neck movement using treats five times twice daily. Rebounding or Standing Rock exercises (Chapter 8) if able to support body weight five times twice daily. Begin facilitated mobilisation for toileting with slings/harnesses. Standing with front legs on physio ball (Chapter 8).

Days 31–45

   Focus for management. Increase mobility. Active range of motion. Increase normal movement through the use of transitions. Proprioceptive retraining. Early strengthening.

   Pain relief. Continue NSAIDS.

   Exercise. 5–10 minutes walking twice daily supported by slings/harness. No games or playing with other dogs. No stairs.

   Modalities. Continue laser and PEMFT at twice-weekly intervals. Once wound healed, introduce hydrotherapy twice weekly. Fill above elbow with water if using UWTM. Go at a slow speed to encourage walking. Gradually increase session intervals from 3 minutes. If in pool, carry out flexion and extension, and weight-shifting exercises on platforms. Again gradually build up length of time in the water and introduce short spells assisted swimming.

Manual therapies. Gentle traction of spine. Conservative gentle mobilisation of stiffened cervical joints.

Therapeutic exercises. Sit to Stand, Down to Sit, Front and Back Leg Lifts, Parastanding with 1 or 2 Books, Scrunchies to The Paw on back legs, Wobble Cushion, Rocker or Wobble Board. Start with five repetitions of exercises twice daily and increase as able. Figures of Eight, five repetitions twice daily (Chapter 8).

Days 46–90

Focus for management. Increase activity levels. Strengthening.

Pain relief. NSAIDS as required.

Exercise. 10–20 minutes walk twice daily and 5 minutes off lead. Start hill work. Low-impact games, such as rolling a ball. No playing with other dogs.

Modalities. Hydrotherapy weekly. Increase depth of water to cover the elbow if using UWTM. Increase speed. If in the pool, introduce free swimming and gradually increase the session interval to 10 minutes.

Therapeutic exercise. Continue exercises as for days 31–45, begin Cavaletti Poles, Dancing, Backwards Walking (Chapter 8). Raise the Cavaletti poles using blocks or drinks cans. Repetitions 10 times twice daily.

Days 91–120

Focus for management. Return to normal activities.

Pain relief. NSAIDS as required.

Exercise. 45 minutes walk twice daily. Off lead for 20 minutes.

Modalities. Hydrotherapy weekly as above.

Therapeutic exercise. As for days 30–60, but increase repetitions by 50%.

Caudal cervical spondylomyelopathy

This usually affects Great Danes (young dogs) and Dobermann Pinschers (much older dogs). One of the authors (DP) has seen very few Dobermann Pinschers presenting in recent years. Protocol is again for a moderate case (Figure 7.32).

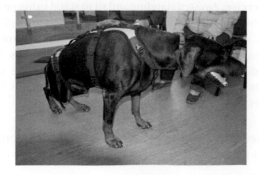

Figure 7.32   A Dobermann Pinscher with caudal cervical spondylomyelopathy.

Signalment. The age of onset can be young (from 3 months) or older 8–9 years. They show signs of neck pain and also may have any of the following: progressive ataxia of back legs, proprioceptive deficits in back legs, short stilted foreleg gait or tetra paresis.

Diagnosis. X-ray with myelogram MRI.

Treatment. Conservative management in cases with mild symptoms or owners who are not looking for surgical management, although surgical management is often recommended.

Surgical Cases Ventral slot, distraction/stabilisation of cervical spine and dorsal laminectomy can all be considered for these cases.

Days 1–14

Focus for management. Wound care, post-operative swelling. Pain control. Bladder and bowel management.

Pain relief. NSAIDS and opiates as required.

Exercise. Strict cage rest with toilet breaks and organised controlled physiotherapy sessions only.

Diet. Advise weight loss if required.

Manual therapies. Massage legs, especially back legs. Vibration and tapping of back leg musculature to encourage contraction.

Modalities. Icing operative site. Twice daily 10 minutes for first 5 days. Laser 3 j/cm^2 at spinal cord. PEMFT set for pain relief (see manufacturers' settings).

Therapeutic exercise. Perform passive ROM of the all legs, five repetitions twice daily. Correct positioning of legs into sitting, lying to promote normal tone. *Do Not Manipulate the Neck.*

Days 15–30

Focus for management. Start gentle movement of neck. Increasing ROM of legs. Begin mobilisation.

Pain relief. NSAIDS. As required.

Exercise. Gradually build up to 5 minutes on level ground in a harness.

Modalities. Laser 3 j/cm^2 at spinal cord. PEMFT set for pain relief (see manufacturers' settings).

Therapeutic exercise. Assisted standing and sit to stand using peanut/slings/hoist/chest harness to support abdomen 2 minutes five times daily or as tolerated by the animal. Active leg withdrawal on tickling feet or gently pinching feet. Slow controlled active head/neck movement using treats five times twice daily. Rebounding or Standing Rock (Chapter 8) if able to support body weight five times twice daily. Begin facilitated mobilisation for toileting with slings/harnesses.

Days 31–45

Focus for management. Increase mobility. Active range of motion. Increase normal movement through the use of transitions. Proprioceptive retraining. Early strengthening.

Pain relief. NSAIDS as required.

Exercise. 5–10 minutes twice daily supported by slings/harness initially, if required. No games or playing with other dogs. No stairs.

Modalities. Continue laser and PEMFT at twice-weekly intervals. Once wound healed, introduce hydrotherapy twice weekly. Just cover the feet with water if using UWTM. Go at a slow speed to encourage active ROM. Gradually increase session intervals from 3 minutes. If in pool, carry out flexion and extension, and weight-shifting exercise on platforms. Again gradually build up length of time in the water and short spells introduce assisted swimming.

Therapeutic exercises. Sit to Stand, Front and Back Leg Lifts, Parastanding 1 or 2 books, Tapping, Scrunchies to Paws on back legs, Wobble Cushion, Rocker or Wobble Board, Front Legs on Swiss Ball (Chapter 8). Start with five repetitions of exercises twice daily and increase as able.

Days 46–60

Focus for management. Increase activity levels. Strengthening.

Pain relief. NSAIDS as required.

Exercise. 10–20 minutes walk twice daily and 5 minutes off lead. Start hill work. Low-impact games, such as rolling a ball. No playing with other dogs.

Modalities. Hydrotherapy weekly. Increase depth of water to cover the elbow if using UWTM. Increase speed. If in the pool, introduce free swimming and gradually increase to 10 minutes.

Therapeutic exercise. Continue exercises as for days 15–30, begin Cavaletti Poles, Figures of Eight, Dancing, Backwards Walking. Raise the Cavaletti poles using blocks or drinks cans. Repetitions 10 times twice daily.

Days 61–90

Focus for management. Return to normal activities.

Pain relief. NSAIDS as required.

Exercise. 45 minutes walk twice daily. Off lead for 20 minutes. Gentle games and playing with other dogs.

Modalities. Hydrotherapy weekly as mentioned above.

Therapeutic exercise. As for days 30–60, but increase repetitions by 50%.

Thoracolumbar intervertebral disc disease (Figure 7.33)

In this disease, disc material prolapses into the spinal canal causing cord compression.

Signalment. The condition is graded 1–5 depending upon severity of clinical signs. Grade 1 dogs show pain with no neurological signs. Grades 2–4 dogs show increasing degrees of back leg ataxia and paresis/paralysis, but are still able to feel deep pain. Grade 5 dogs are paralysed in the back legs and deep pain negative.

Diagnosis. Myelogram, MRI.

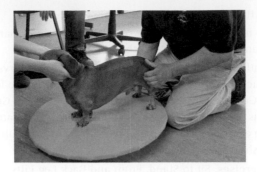

Figure 7.33   Dachshund recovering from thoracolumbar disc protrusion.

Treatment. Surgical decompression and removal of prolapsed disc material.

The suggested rehabilitation is for grades 2–3. Grade 4 dogs will take longer to recover. Grade 5 dogs should follow the protocol initially but consider introducing to a cart at an early stage once bladder and bowl functions are adequately managed. It is also worth considering putting the grade 4 dogs in a cart as a temporary measure. These dogs will fatigue quickly, therefore it is better to conduct short physiotherapy sessions more frequently throughout the day.

Days 1–10

Focus for management. Pain relief. Wound care. Bladder and bowl management.

Pain relief. NSAIDS +/− opiates as required.

Diet. Weight loss as required.

Exercise. Strict cage rest with toilet breaks and controlled physiotherapy sessions only.

Modalities. Icing operative site. 10 minutes twice daily for first 5 days. Laser 3 j/cm^2 at spinal cord. Twice weekly. PEMFT set for pain relief (see manufacturers' settings). Twice weekly. EMS (Chapter 5) 5 minutes twice weekly if FLACCID muscle tone.

Manual Therapies. Mild tail pulls.

Therapeutic exercise. Assisted standing 2 minutes five times daily. Tapping quadriceps and hamstrings if flaccid muscle tone. Icing or flexing to break spasm if hypertonic. Sternal Recumbency/Sphinx Lying. 2 minutes five times daily. Passive ROM of hips, stifles, hock and digits (Chapter 8) three repetitions twice daily.

Days 11–20

Focus for management. Bladder and bowel management as required. Start proprioception retraining. Normalising muscle tone.

Pain relief. NSAIDS as required

Exercise. Still restricted cage rest with toilet breaks.

Modalities. Continue laser and PEMFT twice weekly. Introduce hydrotherapy 4 minutes twice weekly.

Manual therapies. Tail pulls.

Therapeutic exercise. Assisted standing 3 minutes five times daily. Tapping quadriceps and hamstrings if flaccid muscle tone. Icing or flexing to break spasm if hypertonic. Sternal Recumency/Sphinx Lying. 3 minutes five times daily. Transition from lateral recumbency to lying, to sphinx lying to sit to stand, three repetitions five times daily. Passive ROM of hips, stifles, hock and digits five repetitions twice daily. Rebounding 1 minute twice daily. Hair scrunchies to back feet 20 minutes twice daily. Ear and floor scratching 30 seconds of each twice daily.

Days 21–60

Focus for management. Proprioception retraining. Core stability and early strengthening.

Pain relief. NSAIDS as required.

Exercise. 5 minutes initially, building up to 10 minutes twice daily on flat even ground. No games or playing with other dogs.

Modalities. Continue laser and PEMFT twice weekly. Hydrotherapy session intervals gradually building to 10 minutes twice weekly.

Manual therapies. Tail pulls.

Therapeutic exercise. Transition from lateral recumbency to lying, to sphinx lying to sit to stand, five repetitions five times daily. Rebounding 2 minutes twice daily. Hair scrunchies to back feet 20 minutes twice daily. Ear and floor scratching 30 seconds of each twice daily. Unassisted standing starting at 1 minute gradually building to 3 minutes five times daily. Book Standing various arrangements making a total of 4 minutes twice daily. Wobble Board/Cushion starting with 1 minute twice daily building to 4 minutes twice daily. Air Mattress (Chapter 8) starting with 1 minute twice daily building to 5 minutes twice daily.

Days 61–120

Focus for management. Strengthening continued proprioceptive retraining.

Pain relief. NSAIDS as required.

Exercise. Start at 15 minutes twice daily and gradually build up to 30 minutes twice daily. Introduce moderate hills. No games or playing with other dogs.

Modalities. Hydrotherapy session intervals gradually building to 20 minutes weekly.

Therapeutic exercise. Wobble Board/Cushion starting with 5 minutes twice daily. Air Mattress starting with 5 minutes twice daily. Ladder and Obstacle Course five passes twice daily of each. Tug of War high up 10 tugs twice daily. Backwards Walking start with 3 m (10 ft) twice daily and build to 10 m (33 ft) twice daily (Chapter 8).

Lumbosacral disease

This term covers a vast array of possible causes and treatments. The nerve roots are compromised from a variety of causes. Some need surgical intervention with dorsal laminectomy and fenestration of the lumbosacral disc. Some require distraction and fusion of the L7/S1 space. This protocol is for the milder non-surgical cases.

Signalment. Clinical signs can include back leg weakness, ataxia, slow conscious proprioceptive deficits and pain on manipulation of the L/S junction.

Diagnosis. MRI, CT scan.

Treatment. Some milder cases respond well to physiotherapy. We see a lot of bulging L/S discs in agility collies. These dogs are often refusing or measuring jumps. Some will carry one or other back leg intermittently. Dogs with more severe clinical signs will need surgery. More recently we have had good results using shock wave.

Focus for management. Pain relief and mobilisation of the spine.

Pain relief. NSAIDS as required.

Modalities. Laser 12 j/cm^2 at the nerve roots twice weekly. PEMFT set for pain relief (see manufacturers' instructions) twice weekly. Warming of the area before manual therapies is of benefit. We sometimes use ultrasound on a continuous setting 1 MHz, intensity 1.0 W/cm^2 for 5 minutes for a small dog and 10 minutes for a large dog.

Manual therapies. Joint mobilisations to facet joints. Traction (Chapter 6) hold for 15 seconds. Repeat three times twice daily. Tail pulls hold for 15 seconds three times repeated twice daily.

Therapeutic exercise. Biscuits from the Shoulders 10 repetitions twice daily to both sides. Repeat for Biscuts from Ribs, Hips, Toes of Rear Feet, Cat Stretches and Crawl (Chapter 8) again repeated 10 times twice daily. These exercises have the effect of opening up the foramen and mobilising fascial tissue in the area. Flex and extend the spine laterally, dorsally, ventrally and with rotation. Cavaletti Poles, 10 passes twice daily, are also introduced not only because it is a good proprioceptive exercise but also because many of these dogs are pacing.

If there is any muscle wasting, then hydrotherapy, EMS and rear leg strengthening exercises are also used.

Recovery periods vary, but improvement is normally seen within the first 3 weeks. The exercises are carried out indefinitely on a daily basis.

Lower motor neuron disease

Hereditary forms of LMN disease are seen in various breeds and the reader is referred to the further reading section for books listing them.

Acquired acute LMN, for example, polyradiculomyelopathy

This LMN condition usually involves demyelination of the large nerve fibres and is similar to Guillain–Barre syndrome in people. The cause is thought to be immune mediated. These dogs will recover as re-myelination takes place, but this can take many months (Figure 7.34).

Signalment. A single leg can be affected but more often multiple legs are involved. There is paresis or paralysis, loss of reflexes and severe early muscle wasting.

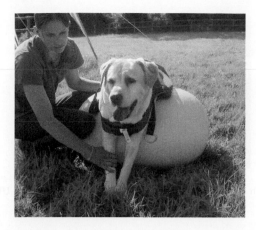

Figure 7.34 A dog with LMN lesion being supported on a peanut while gently taking some of its own weight through the affected front legs.

Diagnosis. Electrodiagnostics, nerve biopsy.

Environment. Avoidance of pressure sores. Ample soft bedding.

Treatment. Trying to work muscles that are very weak is a balance between trying to strengthen without fatiguing.

Therapeutic exercise. Passive ROM to all joints of affected legs three repetitions twice daily. Support dog on peanut ball and gradually lower legs to weight bear. Weight bearing for 20 s. Repeat three times per session, five sessions daily. Use the withdrawal reflex to try to get a muscle contraction. Repeat three times each session. Repeat sessions five times daily. Stimulate muscle contractions by tapping brushing or using a vibrator.

Once these dogs start to show signs of recovery, strengthening exercises such as Sit to Stand and Down to SIt can be introduced. This type of exercise is even better if the dog knew an oral command for the action before it was ill. This way the dog understands what is being asked of it and will try to assist. Assisted standing and transitions from lying to sitting to stand are also being used in recovery. Typically, three repetitions five times daily. Gait retraining is also used for initially five paces repeated five times daily. Once the dog shows signs of good muscle contractions, short hydrotherapy sessions can be introduced. The recovery period can be over 6 months.

Acquired chronic LMN

These are neuropathies seen with conditions such as diabetes mellitus, Cushing's disease and hypothyroidism. There is usually moderate to severe muscle loss and weakness. Treatment is much as for the acute form, but as these are usually older dogs with chronic disease, recovery is incomplete.

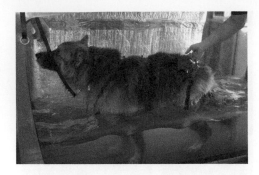

Figure 7.35   GSD with degenerative myelopathy being helped in to the UWTM using a Help 'em up harness.

Degenerative myelopathy (DM) (Figure 7.35)

Sometimes referred to as chronic degenerative reticulomyelopathy (CDRM).

Signalment. Middle age to older large breed dog, usually German Shepherd, showing progressive ataxia of the back legs. Muscle atrophy can be marked. Bowel and bladder functions are usually unaffected.

Diagnosis. Definitive diagnosis is by histology of spinal cord after death. Presumptive diagnosis in the living dog is by ruling out other causes such as disc disease, lumbosacral disease and spinal tumours (MRI). A genetic test is available to identify SOD1 mutation on one or both chromosomes.

Diet. Supplementation with vitamin B complex and B12 in particular, Vitamin E (2000 IU/day), aminocaproic acid and *N*-acetylcystine. Omega 3 fatty acids, coenzyme Q and gamma linoleic acid have all been reported as slowing the rate of deterioration.

Environment. Check flooring and access points. Advise rugs, runners and ramps accordingly.

Pain relief. The condition itself does not appear to be painful, but these dogs will often have other issues such as OA from hip dysplasia that will need pain medication.

Treatment. There is no cure for the condition, but physiotherapy can significantly extend the life spans of these dogs. Aids are of great use in these cases. Treatment is aimed at maintaining muscle mass and nerve stimulation in the back legs. This is a balancing act where it is desirable to work these dogs quite hard but avoid muscle fatigue. Another important consideration is protection of the back feet and nails.

Exercise. 5–10 minute walks five times daily on a variety of terrains. Hill work is encouraged, provided there is no fatigue.

Modalities. Hydrotherapy at least once a week. Session intervals of work and rest building up to 20 minute sessions. In UWTM, a therapist should assist in correct paw placement during the session. If in the pool, then do weight-shifting exercises as well as swimming.

Acupuncture. Start with weekly sessions a monitoring response. Also worth trying electro-acupuncture with or without reversing the polarities.

Manual therapies. Massage. Stroking for 10 minutes followed by kneading of legs and paraspinal muscles for 10 minutes followed by repeating the stroking of the same muscles (Chapter 6).

Therapeutic exercise. Passive ROM, flexion and extension of hips, stifles, hocks and digits three repetitions twice daily. Sit to Stand five repetitions five times daily, Rebounding 1 minute five times daily and Stair Standing 1 minute five times daily (Chapter 8).

Aids. Foot protection. Initially nail guards may be sufficient, but as the condition progresses other types of foot protection will be needed. These range from rubber foot protectors, sciatic slings, to dorsiflex assist boots (Chapter 9).

Harnesses. Two handle harness (Help 'em Up) (Chapter 9) make manoeuvring these dogs much easier for both the patient and the owner.

Carts. All of these dogs will eventually go off their back legs. Many owners may request euthanasia at or before this point. However, many owners may elect to put their dog in a cart. Most dogs adapt extremely well to their newfound mobility and independence. It is imperative that the cart fits the dog. Some carts are custom built, whereas others have multiple adjusting bars. The custom-built carts are more expensive but are able to sustain more wear and tear (Chapter 9).

Fibrocartilaginous embolism

This usually affects young medium to large breed dogs engaging in exercise e.g. Border Collies and Labrador Retrievers. The condition has been reported in smaller breeds, such as Shetland Sheepdogs, Miniature Schnauzers and Yorkshire Terriers.

Signalment. The onset is usually acute following trauma or often dogs jumping whilst exercising so mainly young active dogs are seen. The symptoms are usually strongly lateralised to one side or the other, non-painful and non-progressive (after first 24 hours.) Exact clinical signs, for example, back leg only, back and front leg affected, will depend on the level of the infarct.

Diagnosis. Clinical history, signalment and clinical signs are often enough for diagnosis but early myelogram may show spinal cord swelling or MRI can be more sensitive and will rule out disc extrusion.

Treatment. Conservative management. Prognosis depends on the extent of spinal cord damage determined by the severity of the clinical signs and the amount of immediate functional recovery.

Days 1–14

Focus for management. This depends on the clinical signs that the animal presents with, ranging from high tone to flaccidity. All animals will benefit from proprioceptive work to encourage neural plasticity.

Pain relief. None

Exercise. If non-ambulatory, position legs to encourage elongation of muscles with high tone, supported mobilisation and toileting. In ambulatory patients, short slow walks for 5–10 minutes, supported with slings, if required twice daily.

Diet. Advise weight loss if required.

Environment. Check flooring at home. Advise rugs and runners where appropriate to reduce slipping whilst dog has neurological signs.

Manual therapies. Massage legs especially affected legs. Vibration and tapping to give proprioceptive input. Stretches to prevent contractures forming.

Modalities. Start hydrotherapy twice weekly after first week if ambulatory patient. Fill to above elbows to support the dog in water. Go at a slow speed to encourage walking. Gradually increase session intervals from 3 minutes. If in pool, carry out flexion and extension, and weight-shifting exercises on platforms. Again gradually build up length of time in the water and introduce short spells of assisted swimming.

Therapeutic exercise. In non-ambulatory animal, perform passive ROM to all legs five repetitions twice daily. Correct positioning of legs into sitting, lying to promote normal tone. Assisted standing and sit to stand using peanut/slings/hoist/chest harness to support abdomen 2 minutes five times daily or as tolerated by the animal. Proprioceptive exercises, such as leg withdrawal by tickling feet or gently pinching feet, Mimic Weight Bearing, Rebounding or Standing Rock. if able to support body weight five times twice daily. If ambulatory. Taping or Scrunchie to Paw, Wobble Cushion, Rocker or Wobble Board. Start with five repetitions of exercises twice daily and increase as able (Chapter 8).

Day 15 onwards

Focus for management. If showing signs of functional recovery, increase the amount of normal movement, strengthening and proprioceptive input.

Pain relief. None.

Exercise. Increasing length of walks from 5 minutes supported walks (if originally non-ambulatory) to 20–30 minutes lead walks and 5 minutes off lead.

Modalities. In non-ambulatory patients, start with hydrotherapy as mentioned above. Increase depth of water to cover the elbow if using UWTM. Increase speed. If in the pool, introduce free swimming and gradually increase to 10 minutes.

Manual therapies. Stretching to prevent contractures where appropriate.

Therapeutic exercise. Continue proprioceptive work Wobble Cushion, Rocker or Wobble Board, Cavaletti Poles, Figures of Eight, Standing with Front Legs on Swiss Ball, Parastanding, Dancing and Backwards Walking (Chapter 8). Raise the Cavaletti poles using blocks or drinks cans. Introduce strengthening exercises such as walking downhill. Start with 10 repetitions of exercises twice daily and increase as able.

CHAPTER 8
Therapeutic exercise

Therapeutic exercise is the basis of physiotherapy treatment. It is the most important part of the rehabilitation programme. A home exercise programme gives owners a chance to feel very involved in their animal's rehabilitation and it means that a therapeutic intervention can occur every day. As home exercises form the basis of the rehabilitation, it is very important that time is spent in teaching the owner how to correctly perform the exercises, and the provision of pictures will aid compliance.

We use exercise to prepare the body for specific performance events, rehabilitate after injury or improve health/well-being/fitness and we need to be aware of the specific goals for completing the exercise. This will influence the type of exercise to be utilised. Exercise can be placed into broad categories: Active or passive range of movement (ROM); strength and endurance. For exercise to cause a change, the muscles or joints have to be overloaded. Exercises must be specific to the animal they are being prescribed for; an exercise for a fit agility dog is unlikely to be appropriate for an elderly overweight arthritic dog. The exercise needs to be of an appropriate intensity, duration and frequency to overload the dog and cause a change in muscle, however not to go beyond its physical capability.

The exercises demonstrated in this chapter have the number of repetitions attached to them. This is to give the reader an idea of the number of repetitions commonly used. However, these should be altered for each patient based on clinical examination.

Tip: The exercises with a space left for the number of repetitions can be downloaded from www.physio-vet.com. Enter the code on the inside cover of this book to gain access to these downloads.

The exercises are listed under the heading of ROM, core stability, proprioception, strength and endurance so that they can be easily referred to. However, many of the exercises can be used for dual purposes. For example, walking over poles can be an active ROM exercise or a strengthening exercise for the front or back legs, a scrunchie on the nose improves front leg ROM and strengthens but also increases weight bearing on the backleg and using leg weights or cuffs will increase strength and proprioception of that leg.

Range of movement

ROM is an essential requirement for movement to take place. ROM is classified into inner/mid and outer ranges. Inner range is where the muscle moving the joint is fully

Practical Physiotherapy for Small Animal Practice, First Edition.
Edited by David Prydie and Isobel Hewitt.
© 2015 John Wiley & Sons, Ltd. Published 2015 by John Wiley & Sons, Ltd.
Companion Website: www.wiley.com/go/practical-physiotherapy-for-small-animals

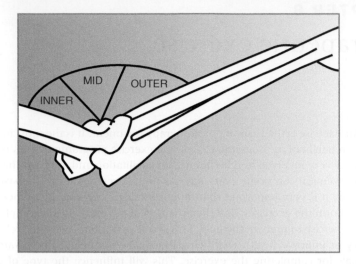

Figure 8.1 *Joint range of movement.* The motion of a joint can occur through inner, mid and outer range of motion. Passive ROM.

contracted and the bones are at the limit of their movement. Outer range is where the muscle moving the joint is at full stretch and the bones are at the limit of their movement in the opposite direction (Figure 8.1). ROM is affected by joint surfaces, articular cartilage, joint capsule and ligaments. In animals with degenerative joint disease, it may be that we can improve the ROM so it becomes functional but not able to restore full normal ROM often due to bony exotoses. Increased ROM can cause as much pain as reduced ROM as it is caused by increased laxity in the joint capsule and ligaments (hypermobility). It is inadvisable to do passive ROM exercises in these animals (Chapter 6 describes passive ROM technique). When working to increase ROM, the exercises should be started in the inner range and worked out further into the outer range as ROM increases. Passive and active exercises can increase ROM, and increased range can be enhanced if the joints are warmed before exercise. This is due to the relaxation of the joint capsules and ligaments.

Examples of passive ROM exercises
Passive exercises are important especially when the animal is unable to move the joints voluntarily. PROM exercises will not affect muscle mass, strength or endurance, and therefore they should be progressed to active exercises as early as possible. This will improve ROM, but also start training neuromuscular control and muscle strength (Figures 8.2–8.26).

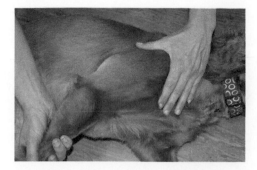

Figure 8.2 *Shoulder flexion*. With the dog lying on its side, gently bring the upper foreleg back towards the rear leg. Try to have the elbow pointing to the spine. Hold for 10–15 seconds. Repeat three times twice daily.

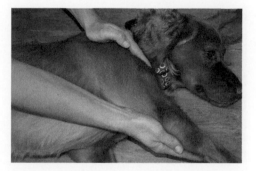

Figure 8.3 *Shoulder extension*. With the dog lying on its side, gently bring the upper foreleg forwards towards its nose. Try to have the elbow straight. Hold for 10–15 seconds. Repeat three times twice daily.

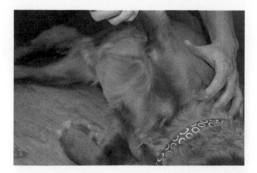

Figure 8.4 *Shoulder abduction*. With the dog lying on its side, gently grasp below the elbow and bring the leg up towards the ceiling. Stabilise the scapular to prevent it lifting. Hold for 10–15 seconds. Repeat three times twice daily.

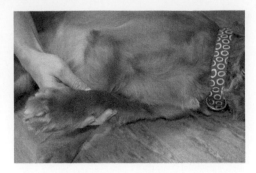

Figure 8.5 *Shoulder adduction.* With the dog lying on its side and on the affected leg, gently grasp below the elbow and bring the leg up towards the ceiling. Hold for 10–15 seconds. Repeat three times twice daily.

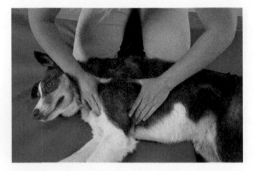

Figure 8.6 *Scapular mobilisations.* With the dog lying on its side, grasp around the caudal and cranial borders of the scapula. Gently move the scapula forwards, backwards, up and down. Repeat for 30 seconds. Repeat three times twice daily.

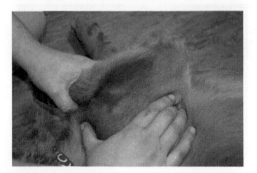

Figure 8.7 *Elbow flexion.* With the dog lying on its side, place one hand behind the elbow and upper part of the leg. Gently bring the lower part of the leg towards the head. Hold for 10–15 seconds. Repeat three times twice daily.

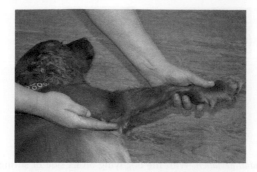

Figure 8.8 *Elbow extension*. With the dog lying on its side, place one hand behind the elbow and upper part of the leg. Gently bring the lower part of the leg away from the head as if trying to straighten the elbow. Hold for 10–15 seconds. Repeat three times twice daily.

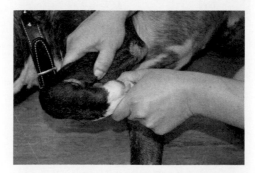

Figure 8.9 *Carpal flexion*. With the dog lying on its side, gently bring the paw towards the back of the leg so that the pads get as close to the leg as possible. Hold for 10–15 seconds. Repeat three times twice daily.

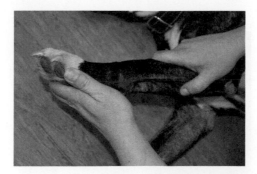

Figure 8.10 *Carpal extension*. With the dog lying on its side, hold the leg above the carpus (wrist) and gently push the foot forward so that the leg straightens. Hold for 10–15 seconds. Repeat three times twice daily.

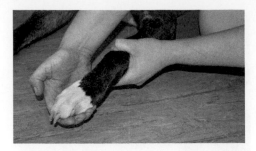

Figure 8.11   *Carpal radial deviation.* With the dog lying on its side or sitting, grasp the foreleg above the carpus to stabilise it. Holding the carpus in neutral with one hand, hold the paw with the other hand and move it towards midline. Hold for 10–15 seconds. Repeat three times twice daily.

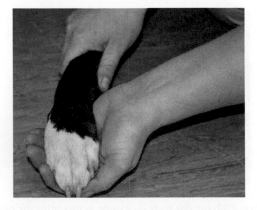

Figure 8.12   *Carpal ulnar deviation.* With the dog lying on its side or sitting, grasp the foreleg above the carpus to stabilise it. Holding the carpus in neutral with one hand, hold the paw with the other hand and move it away from midline. Hold for 10–15 seconds. Repeat three times twice daily.

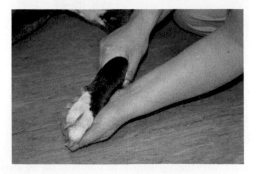

Figure 8.13   *Carpal supination.* With the dog lying on its side or sitting, grasp the foreleg above the carpus to stabilise it. Hold the paw on the outside border and turn the paw rotating it inwards. Hold for 10–15 seconds. Repeat three times twice daily.

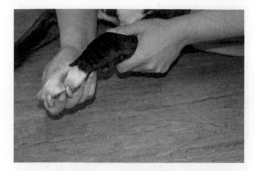

Figure 8.14   *Carpal pronation.* With the dog lying on its side or sitting, grasp the foreleg above the carpus to stabilise it. Hold the paw on the inside border and turn the paw rotating it outwards. Hold for 10–15 seconds. Repeat three times twice daily.

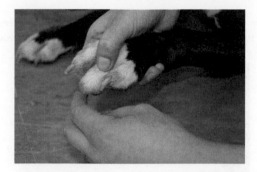

Figure 8.15   *Digit flexion.* Hold the toe by the nail and gently bend towards the pad. Hold for 10–15 seconds. Repeat three times twice daily. Repeat for each toe.

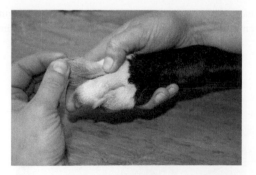

Figure 8.16   *Digit extension.* Hold the toe by the nail and gently pull upwards. Hold for 10–15 seconds. Repeat three times twice daily. Repeat for each toe.

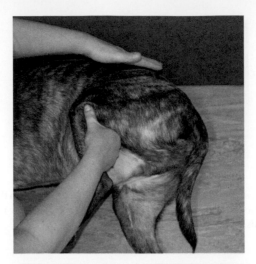

Figure 8.17 *Hip flexion.* With the dog lying on its side, grasp above the knee and bring the knee forwards towards the head. Hold for 10–15 seconds. Repeat three times twice daily.

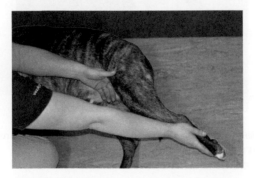

Figure 8.18 *Hip extension.* With the dog lying on its side, grasp the leg and gently bring backwards. Try to straighten the knee. Hold for 10–15 seconds. Repeat three times twice daily.

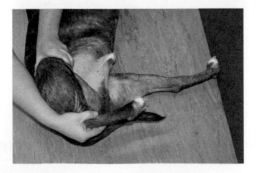

Figure 8.19 *Hip abduction.* With the dog lying on its side, hold the affected leg above the stifle and gently lift the leg upwards away from the midline of its body. Hold for 10–15 seconds. Repeat three times twice daily.

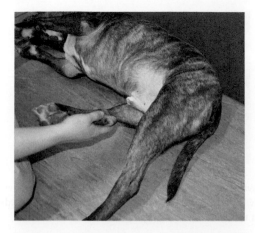

Figure 8.20 *Hip adduction.* With the dog lying on its affected side, grasp the lower leg and gently lift upwards towards the ceiling. Hold for 10–15 seconds. Repeat three times twice daily.

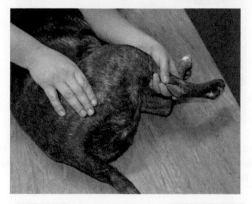

Figure 8.21 *Stifle flexion.* With the dog lying on its side, grasp the leg above the knee with one hand. Grasp the hock with the other hand and bring the hock towards the dog's bottom. Hold for 10–15 seconds. Repeat three times twice daily.

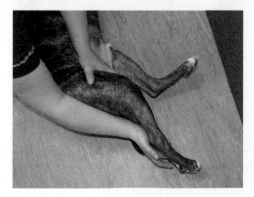

Figure 8.22 *Stifle extension.* With the dog lying on its side, place one hand on the front of the thigh. Grasp the leg above the hock with the other hand and move the lower part of the leg forward as if straightening the stifle. Hold for 10–15 seconds. Repeat three times twice daily.

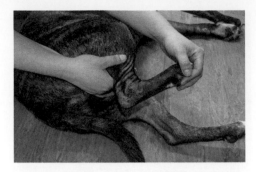

Figure 8.23 *Hock flexion.* With the dog lying on its side, grasp the leg above the hock with one hand. Grasp the foot with the other hand and move the foot gently towards the body. Hold for 10–15 seconds. Repeat three times twice daily.

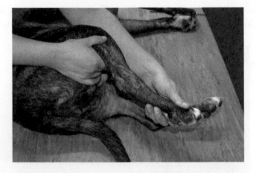

Figure 8.24 *Hock extension.* With the dog lying on its side, grasp the leg above the hock with one hand. Grasp the foot with the other hand and move the foot backwards. Hold for 10–15 seconds. Repeat three times twice daily.

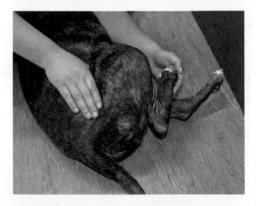

Figure 8.25 *Simulated sitting.* With the dog lying on its side, gently grasp the front of the thigh with one hand. Place the flat of the other hand on the pads of the foot and gently push towards the other hand. The ankle (hock) and knee (stifle) should flex as if sitting. Hold this position for 10–15 seconds. Repeat three times twice daily.

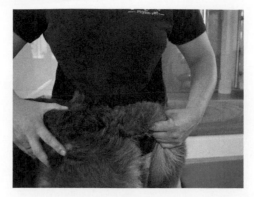

Figure 8.26   *Tail circles.* Hold the pelvis and stabilise with one hand, with the other hand grasp the tail approximately 5 cm (2 inches) from the base and create a gentle curve. Rotate the tail clockwise and anticlockwise. Repeat 10 times each way twice daily.

Examples of active ROM exercises

The amount of ROM can also be affected by the flexibility of the soft tissues around the joint. Muscle stiffness and adaptive shortening of the muscle and tendon tissue following injury will reduce the amount of movement available. Stretching of the affected muscles will allow the joint to move through full range (Figures 8.27–8.48).

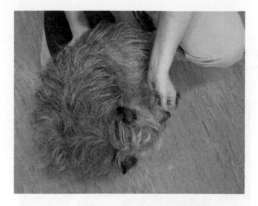

Figure 8.27   *Biscuits to the shoulder.* With the dog standing, move a treat from in front of the dog's nose to the left shoulder. Allow the dog to take the treat. Repeat for the right shoulder. Do 10 repetitions to both shoulders twice daily.

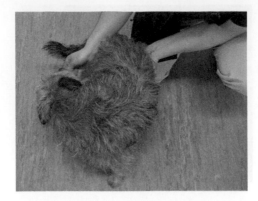

Figure 8.28 *Biscuits to the ribs.* With the dog in standing, take a treat from in front of its nose and move round to over the left rib cage. Allow the dog to take the treat. Repeat for the right rib cage. Do 10 repetitions to each side twice daily.

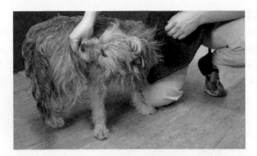

Figure 8.29 *Biscuits from the hips.* With the dog standing, move a treat from the nose to the left hip. Repeat to the right hip. Make sure the dog shifts its weight from side to side. Repeat 10 times twice daily for both sides.

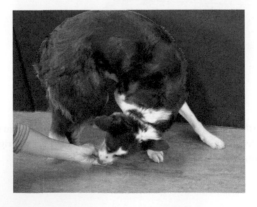

Figure 8.30 *Biscuits from the toes.* With the dog standing, move a treat from the nose to the left hind foot. Repeat to the right hind foot. Make sure the dog shifts its weight from side to side. Repeat 10 times twice daily for both sides.

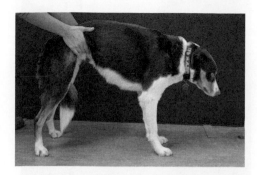

Figure 8.31   *Thoracic lumbar flexion.* With the dog standing, place your fingers on its midline and run your fingers from its chest to the groin to encourage the dog to lift its abdomen. Repeat 10 times twice daily.

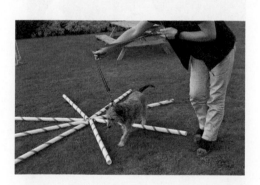

Figure 8.32   *Clock face.* Arrange 1 m length plastic poles (plumbing waste pipes or garden canes/tools) in a clock-face manner. Slowly walk your dog over the poles five times clockwise. Repeat five times anticlockwise. Repeat twice daily.

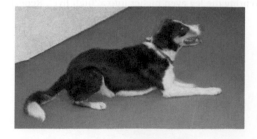

Figure 8.33   *Down to a sit.* Starting with the dog in the down position and call to a sit.

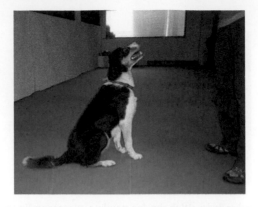

Figure 8.34 *Down to sit.* Give the 'sit' command and have your dog come into a sitting position. Now return to the down position with the 'down' command. Reward. Repeat 10 times twice daily.

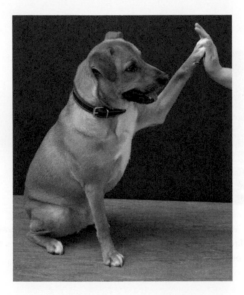

Figure 8.35 *High five.* With the dog in a sitting position, give the 'paw' command. Using a treat, encourage your dog to bring the leg even higher into a 'high five'. Repeat 10 times twice daily on both front legs.

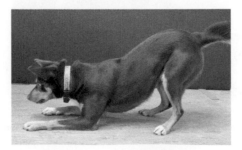

Figure 8.36 *Play bow.* Hold a treat in front of the dog's nose and gently lower the treat to the floor bringing the dog into a play bow position. Reward and repeat 10 times twice daily.

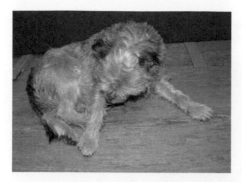

Figure 8.37 *Cream cheese to axilla.* With the dog lying on its side with the affected leg uppermost, place a smear of cream cheese in your dog's armpit. Allow the dog to lick it away. Repeat three times twice daily. Repeat for the other front leg if both sides are affected.

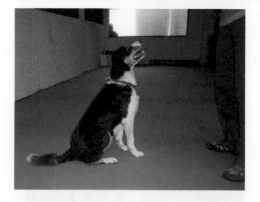

Figure 8.38 *Sit to stand.* Start with the dog in the sitting position and call to a stand.

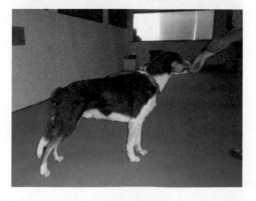

Figure 8.39 *Sit to stand.* Give the 'stand' command and have the dog stand on all four legs. Return to the sitting position. Repeat 10 times twice daily.

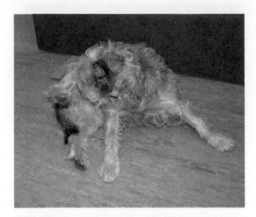

Figure 8.40 *Cream cheese to groin*. With the dog in a lying position and with the affected leg upper most, smear some cream cheese in the dog's groin. Allow the dog to lick it away. Repeat three times twice daily. Repeat for the other back leg if both sides are affected.

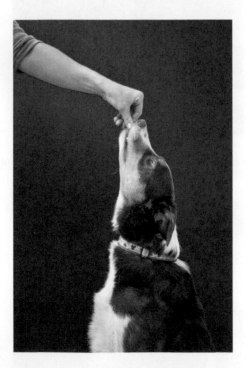

Figure 8.41 *Neck extension*. With the dog in a sitting position, use a treat in a lifting motion above the dog's nose to encourage it to look upwards. Keeping the treat close to the nose as too far away may encourage the dog to jump up. Repeat 10 times twice daily.

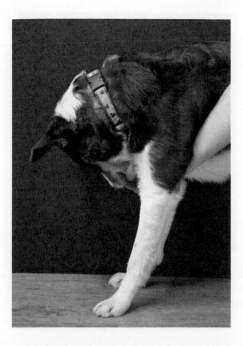

Figure 8.42 *Neck flexion.* With the dog sitting or standing, use a treat to bring its head towards its chest so that it looks down. Repeat 10 times twice daily.

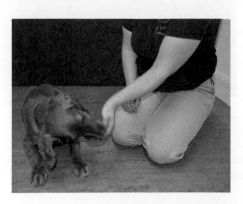

Figure 8.43 *Neck rotation.* With the dog sitting or standing, use a treat in a circular motion away from the dog's nose so that the dog has to turn its head. Repeat 10 times twice daily.

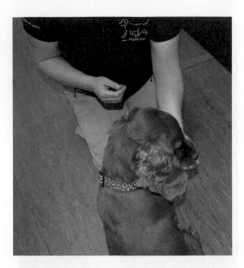

Figure 8.44 *Neck side flexion.* With the dog sitting or standing, use a treat to lure the dog's nose towards its shoulder. Ensure you keep the treat close to the dog's nose so that the dog only moves its neck and not the thoracic spine. Repeat 10 times twice daily.

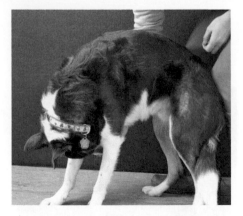

Figure 8.45 *Thoracic and lumbar flexion.* With the dog sitting or standing, use a treat to draw the dog's nose towards its belly. Repeat 10 times twice daily.

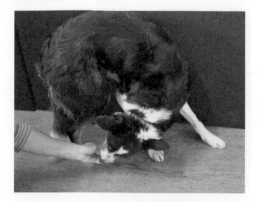

Figure 8.46 *Thoracic side flexion*. With rotation. With the dog standing, use a treat to draw the dog towards its back paw/toes. Repeat to the left or right 10 times twice daily.

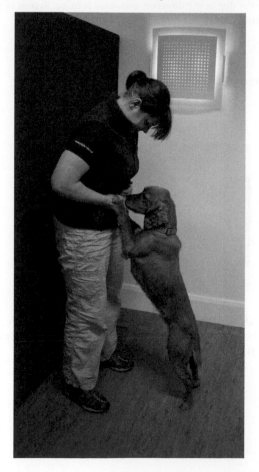

Figure 8.47 *Lumbar extension*. Encourage the dog to jump up and rest its paws on your knees, waist, chest or shoulders, depending upon its size and the amount of extension it can manage. Repeat 10 times twice daily.

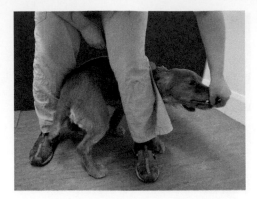

Figure 8.48 *Lumbar side flexion.* With the dog standing and you standing with your legs open, use a treat to encourage the dog to walk in a circle around your leg. Use the hand without the treat in to help guide the dog in the direction you want it to go. Repeat to the other direction as required 10 times twice daily.

Examples of stretches (Figures 8.49–8.54)

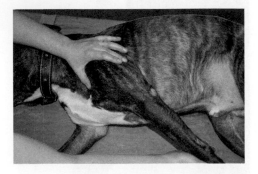

Figure 8.49 *Bicep stretch.* With the dog lying on its side with the affected leg upwards, hold the scapula to stabilise it and bring the leg backwards, flexing the shoulder and extending the elbow. Hold for 20–30 seconds. Repeat three times twice daily.

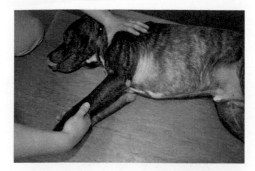

Figure 8.50 *Teres stretch*. With the dog lying on its side with the affected leg upwards, hold the scapula to stabilise it and bring the leg forwards, up towards the ceiling and rotate the paw towards the dog's nose. Hold for 20–30 seconds. Repeat three times twice daily.

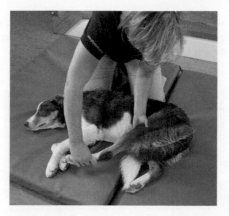

Figure 8.51 *Hamstring stretch*. With the dog lying on its side with the affected side upwards, bring the leg forwards towards the dog's head keeping the stifle straight. Hold for 20–30 seconds. Repeat three times twice daily.

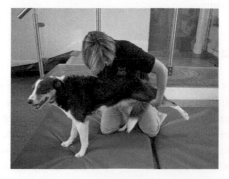

Figure 8.52 *Iliopsoas stretch*. With the dog lying on its side with the affected side upwards or standing, bring the leg backwards, extending the hip. Be careful to keep the spine slightly flexed or in neutral. Hold for 20–30 seconds. Repeat three times twice daily.

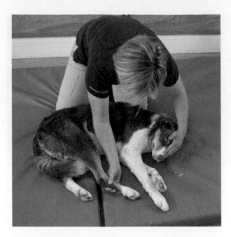

Figure 8.53 *Sciatic nerve stretch.* With the dog lying on its side with the affected side upwards, flex the head towards the chest and bring the affected leg forward keeping the stifle straight. Hold for 10–15 seconds. Repeat three times twice daily.

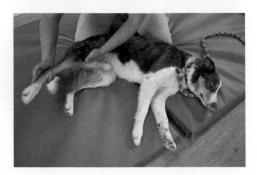

Figure 8.54 *Gracilis stretch.* With the dog lying on its side with the affected leg upwards, bring the leg forward. Keep the stifle straight and lift the leg toward the ceiling. Hold for 20–30 seconds. Repeat three times twice daily.

Core stability and proprioception

Core stability describes the muscles around the trunk and is the basis of all leg activities and movement. Stability of the proximal joints, such as the hip and shoulder, is also vital for leg movement. Good stability of the joints also requires good proprioception and these together will prevent injury. If the muscles that stabilise the joints are weak, the joint will have poor stability leading to abnormal joint movement. The muscles that mobilise the joint will compensate clamping down to act as splint.

Dynamic joint stability is achieved by regulation of muscle tone, intact proprioception and neuromuscular control.

Proprioception is the unconscious perception of joint movement and position. Proprioceptive information is received by the brain or spinal cord from joint mechanoreceptors, muscle spindles and golgi tendon organs. Joint position sense is required for posture and balance, and is also influenced by the visual and vestibular systems. Joint effusion has been shown to reduce the nerve impulses from joint receptors that in turn results in inhibition of muscles that will reduce the stability around a joint. This increases the likelihood of injury or further damage occurring. Central nervous system damage can also alter proprioception. In animals with disc disease, often their conscious proprioception is damaged. As a result, a leg may be put into an abnormal position, such as full abduction, whilst standing and the animal will not be able to move the leg back to the correct position.

Following an injury, proprioception exercises should always be included in the rehabilitation program. These exercises may be simple, such as standing in a normal position on an uneven surface. Standing itself can be a difficult exercise following neurological injury as it requires neuromuscular control and coordination to maintain postural balance and leg position. It is important when retraining proprioception that the exercises have multiple sensory inputs. The exercises can then be progressed by increasing speed, changing surface, reducing the base of support or adding perturbations. Examples of this are starting with assisted standing (Figure 8.56), then moving onto three-leg standing (Figure 8.61), para standing (Figure 8.63) and a wobble cushion (Figure 8.82). The dog can be progressed from rocker boards (Figure 8.83) to wobble boards (Figure 8.84) and standing on a physio ball (Figure 8.68).

Examples of basic core stability or weight-bearing exercises (Figures 8.55–8.65).

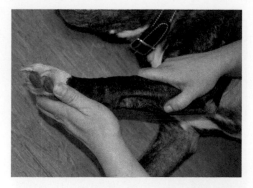

Figure 8.55 *Mimic weight bearing.* With the dog lying on its side, straighten the elbow with one hand. Place the other hand flat on the pads of the dog's paw. Keep the wrist (carpus) straight. Apply gentle pressure. Hold for 10–15 seconds. Repeat three times twice daily.

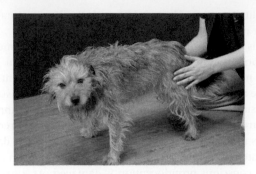

Figure 8.56 *Assisted standing.* Gently support the dog in the standing position. Rock very gently from side to side and back to front. These should be very small movements and should not make the dog move its paws. Continue for 30 seconds. Repeat three times twice daily.

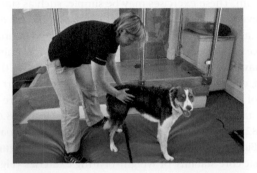

Figure 8.57 *Standing rock.* With the dog standing, making sure it bears weight equally on all four legs. Hold the dog around its hips and gently rock it forwards and backwards. Be careful that you do not push the dog over. Repeat 10 times twice daily.

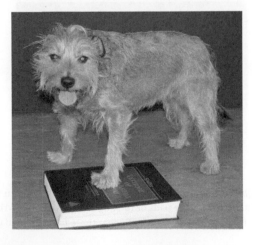

Figure 8.58 *Para standing one book.* Place a book on the floor. Place the dog's paw of the affected leg on the book. Hold for 60 seconds. Repeat three times twice daily. Repeat for any other affected legs.

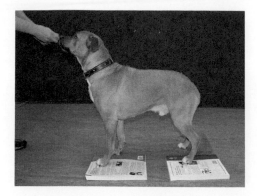

Figure 8.59   *Para standing two books.* Place two books of equal height on the floor. Place the dog's two left feet on the books. Hold for 60 seconds. Repeat three times twice daily. Repeat for the two right feet.

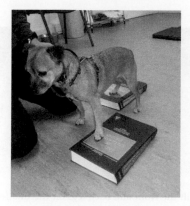

Figure 8.60   *Diagonal book standing.* Place two books of equal height on the floor. Place the dog's two left feet on the books. Hold for 60 seconds. Repeat three times twice daily. Repeat for the two right feet.

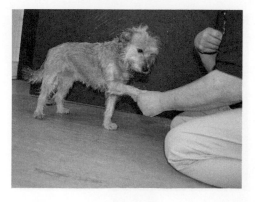

Figure 8.61   *Three-leg standing front leg.* Lift the unaffected front leg of the dog off the ground and hold for 60 seconds or as long as it will tolerate. Repeat three times twice daily. If both front legs are affected, repeat with the other leg.

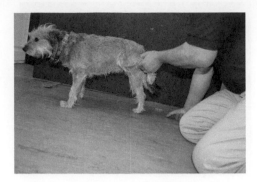

Figure 8.62 *Three-leg standing back leg.* Lift the unaffected back leg of the dog off the ground and hold for 60 seconds or as long as it will tolerate. Repeat three times twice daily. If both back legs are affected, repeat with the other leg.

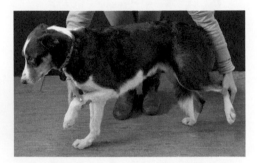

Figure 8.63 *Para standing.* Lift the front and back legs on the unaffected side of the dog. Hold for 60 seconds or as long as it can manage. Repeat three times twice daily. If legs on both sides are affected, repeat with the opposite front and back legs.

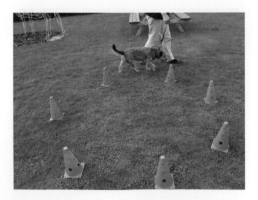

Figure 8.64 *Circles.* Place objects to make a circle. Slowly walk your dog round the circle five times clockwise and anticlockwise. Repeat twice daily.

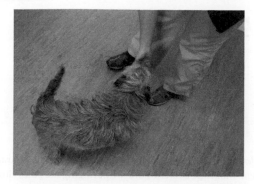

Figure 8.65 *Spins*. With the dog standing, use a treat to encourage it to turn slightly. This can be varied by moving the dog clockwise or anticlockwise and by moving the dog slowly or quickly. Try to ensure the dog does bear weight fully on the affected leg. Repeat 10 times twice daily.

Examples of advanced core stability exercises (Figures 8.66–8.73).

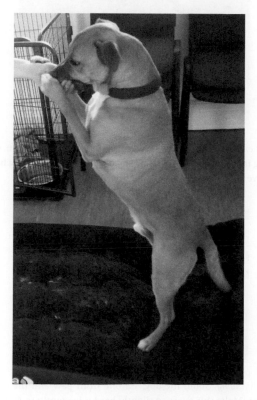

Figure 8.66 *Standing on air mattress*. Standing on an air mattress, use a treat to encourage the dog to come up onto its back legs. Repeat 10 times twice daily.

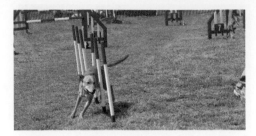

Figure 8.67   *Weave poles.* Place objects or weave poles in a line and encourage the dog to move in and out through them. Make the exercise harder by bringing the poles closer together. Repeat 10 times twice daily.

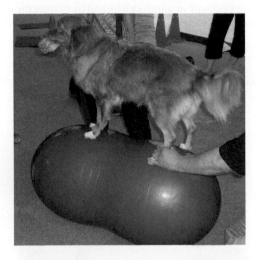

Figure 8.68   *Standing on a Swiss ball.* Place the dog in a standing position on a Swiss ball (or peanut). Hold the dog initially and slowly remove your support as the dog balances. Hold up to 30 seconds. Repeat five times twice daily.

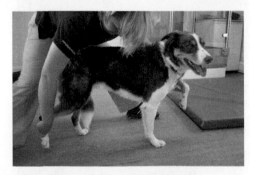

Figure 8.69   *Cross leg standing.* Stand the dog, lift one front paw and the opposite rear leg. Do not lift the affected leg. Make this exercise slightly harder by gently rocking the dog whilst it is standing. Hold up to 30 seconds. Repeat five times twice daily.

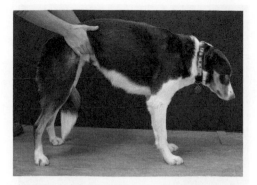

Figure 8.70 *Tummy tickles.* With the dog standing, tickle them underneath its tummy to encourage the dog to lift it. Repeat 10 times twice daily.

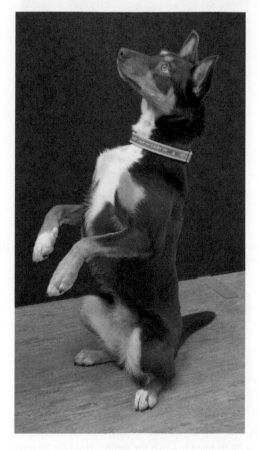

Figure 8.71 *Beg.* Start with the dog sitting and use a treat above its nose to encourage the dog to lift the front legs off the ground. Repeat 10 times twice daily.

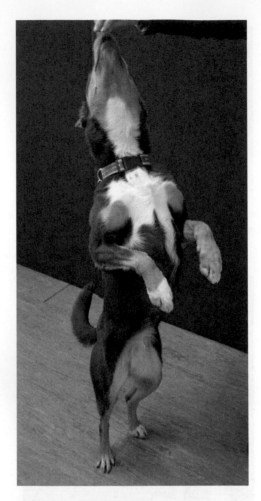

Figure 8.72 *Beg to stand.* Start with the dog in a beg position and use the treat to encourage it to stand up onto its back legs by pushing upwards.

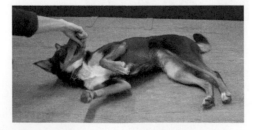

Figure 8.73 *Side sit-ups.* With the dog lying on its side with the affected side upwards, use a treat to encourage the dog to lift its head towards the ceiling. Hold for 10 seconds. Repeat five times twice daily.

Examples of proprioceptive exercises (Figures 8.74–8.86).

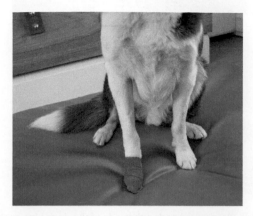

Figure 8.74   *Taping paw.* Using vet wrap or tape, tape around the affected paw. This will prevent the toes splaying and encourage weight bearing. Place on the dog's paw for short intervals and supervise whilst tape is in situ. Repeat twice daily.

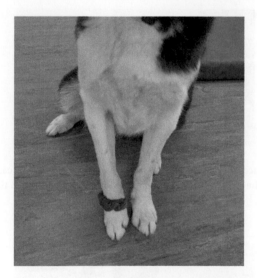

Figure 8.75   *Scrunchie to paw.* Place a hair scrunchie around the affected leg. This will encourage the dog to lift the leg and kick the scrunchie off. Place the scrunchie around the unaffected leg to encourage the dog to bear weight more on the affected leg. Try for short intervals and supervise whilst scrunchie is in situ. Repeat twice daily.

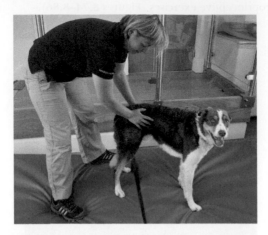

Figure 8.76 *Rebounding.* Place your hands either side of the dog's hips or shoulders and gently push from side to side for 60 seconds. Repeat twice daily. The force should be sufficient to make the dog transfer weight from side to side but not strong enough to knock the dog over.

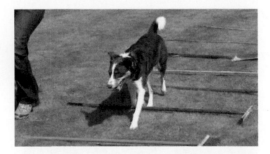

Figure 8.77 *Poles.* Place eight poles or garden canes or tools in a line. Measure the dog to the shoulder. Make this the distance between the poles. Walk the dog through the course five times twice daily.

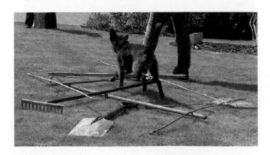

Figure 8.78 *Pick-a-sticks.* Arrange garden tools or canes in 'pick-a-sticks' manner. Walk the dog through the obstacle course 10 times twice daily.

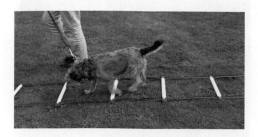

Figure 8.79   *Ladder.* Slowly walk the dog through a step ladder. Repeat five times twice daily.

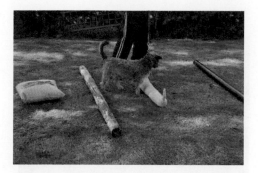

Figure 8.80   *Obstacle course.* Arrange various objects of varying height and width to make an obstacle course. Walk the dog through the course five times twice daily.

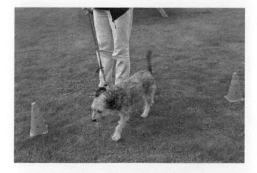

Figure 8.81   *Figures of eight.* Place two objects about three times the height of the dog apart. Slowly walk the dog in a figure of eight manner around the objects. Repeat five times twice daily.

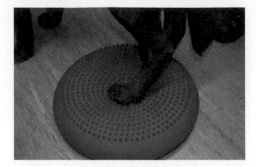

Figure 8.82 *Wobble cushion.* Place the paw of the affected leg on the air cushion or hot water bottle full of air. Hold for 60 seconds or as long as the dog can manage. Repeat three times twice daily. Repeat for any other affected legs.

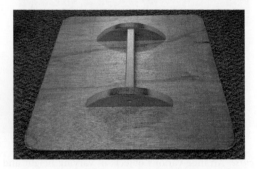

Figure 8.83 *Rocker board.* These are balance boards that only have one direction of movement that the dog can stand on and then progress onto a wobble board.

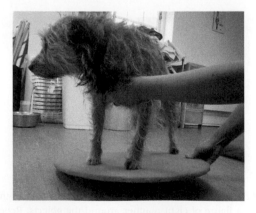

Figure 8.84 *Wobble board.* These are multidirectional balance boards. Stand the dog on the board and move the board to improve weight bearing on the affected leg. Repeat 10 times twice daily.

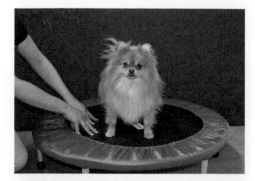

Figure 8.85 *Standing on a trampet.* Stand the dog on a trampet and ensure it is weight bearing through all four legs. Bounce the trampet to challenge standing balance. Repeat 10 times twice daily.

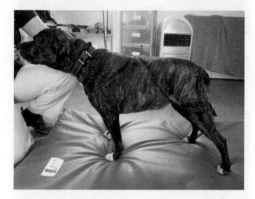

Figure 8.86 *Uneven surface walking.* Place the dog on an uneven surface, such as an air mattress, uneven ground, long grass or sand. Walk for 2 minutes. Repeat twice daily.

Strengthening

Muscle strength is the ability of a muscle to contract maximally to produce the maximum amount of force. A muscular contraction can be influenced by several factors such as the size of the muscle in terms of diameter, the muscle tension/length relationship and the recruitment of motor units. There are different types of con-traction – concentric, eccentric and isometric (where the fibres do not change their length). Concentric contractions are where the muscle fibres are shortening. An example of this is contraction of the biceps as the elbow flexes. Eccentric contractions are where the muscle fibres lengthen. An example of this is the hamstrings length-ening as the animal sits. Isometric exercises will activate stability muscles and can be used when the animal has a limited ROM. They are, therefore, often used as basic strengthening exercises before progressing to concentric and eccentric exercises.

There are numerous ways of increasing the strength of a muscle. This can be done by using resistance, gravity, bodyweight and by adding weights to overload the muscle.

Examples of front leg-strengthening exercises (Figures 8.87–8.95).

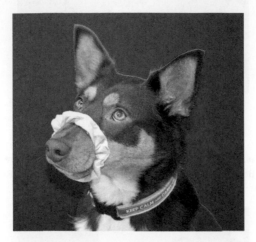

Figure 8.87   *Scrunchie on the nose.* Place a hair scrunchie on the dog's nose (ensure it is not too tight) and encourage the dog to remove the scrunchie with its paws. Repeat 10 times twice daily.

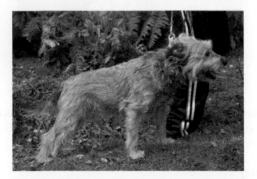

Figure 8.88   *Uphill walking.* Walk the dog slowly up a moderate hill for 5 minutes. Repeat twice daily.

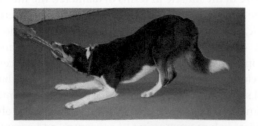

Figure 8.89   *Tug of war low down.* Using a tug toy, have your dog tug vigorously for 30 seconds. Make sure the tug is below the dog's head. Repeat 10 times twice daily. NOTE: This exercise is not suitable for aggressive dogs.

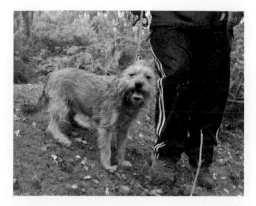

Figure 8.90   *Downhill walking.* Have the dog walk slowly down a moderate hill for 5 minutes. Repeat twice daily.

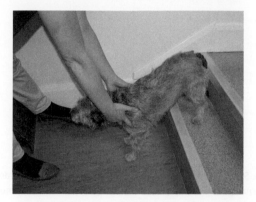

Figure 8.91   *Step down front legs.* On some stairs, have the dog take one or two steps down depending upon size. The front legs should be below the back legs. Hold this position for 60 seconds or as long as the dog can stand. Repeat three times twice daily.

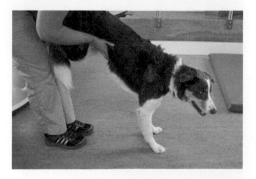

Figure 8.92   *Wheelbarrow.* With the dog standing, hold the dog around its abdomen and lift the rear legs off the ground. Progress the exercise by encouraging the dog to step forwards. Hold for 10–15 seconds. Repeat five times twice daily.

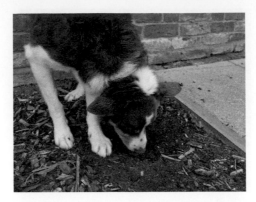

Figure 8.93 *Digging*. Give the dog a designated area or use a sand pit, place a treat or toy in the soil (or sand) and encourage it to dig for 5 minutes. Repeat twice daily.

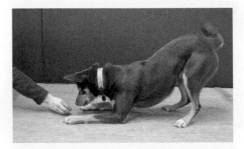

Figure 8.94 *Push-ups*. Start with the dog standing, use a treat to lure the dog down into a play bow position and encourage the dog to push back up again. Repeat 10 times twice daily.

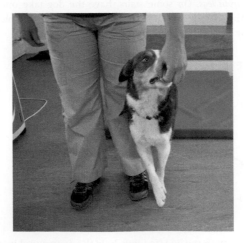

Figure 8.95 *Side stepping*. Start with the dog standing and step towards the dog encouraging it to step away from you. Repeat 10 times twice daily.

Many dogs adopt pacing as an abnormal gait pattern after injury. This should be corrected. Using poles in a straight line will help with gait retraining. The eight poles are used and placed one shoulder height apart (measure the dog from floor to shoulder). Trot the dog over the poles and a normal gait pattern should be adopted. As the dog progresses, one pole can be randomly removed from the sequence and placed at the end. Continue to remove the poles until all the poles are double spaced.

Resistance band or tubing can be used for strengthening and also to increase body awareness. The band is tied around the chest area (or can be attached to a harness if it is not appropriate to be tied around the chest) and crossed underneath the abdominal area. This will engage the abdominal muscles. Then the tubing is brought up and over the gluteal muscles and hamstrings to activate these.

Examples of backleg-strengthening exercises (Figures 8.96–8.108).

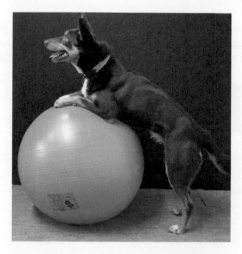

Figure 8.96 *Standing with front legs on a Swiss ball.* Using an appropriate-size ball for the dog's size, stabilise the ball and lift the dog's front legs onto the ball so it is supported under its chest. Gently rock the ball backwards and forwards. Repeat for a minute. Repeat five times twice daily.

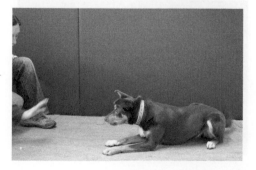

Figure 8.97 *Crawl.* With the dog in a down position, use a treat to lure it forwards. You can also encourage a dog to crawl by placing an obstacle such as a jump or agility tunnel and lure it underneath. Repeat 10 times twice daily.

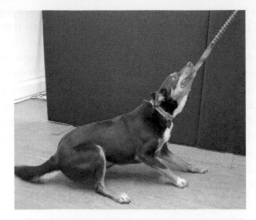

Figure 8.98 *Tug of war high up.* Use a tug toy and encourage the dog to pull on the toy. Make sure the toy is being tugged from above the dog's head. This will produce thrust on the back legs. Repeat five times twice daily. NOTE: This exercise is not suitable for aggressive dogs.

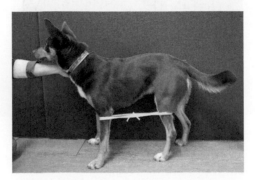

Figure 8.99 *Resisted walking.* This can be used for front or rear leg strengthening. Tie the band in a loop around the dog's legs, above the elbow and encourage the dog to walk for 5 minutes twice daily.

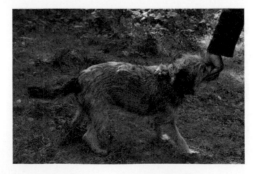

Figure 8.100 *Backwards walking.* Hold a treat at your dog's face and gently push towards the nose encouraging your dog to walk backwards. Try to manage 3 metres at a time. Repeat three times twice daily.

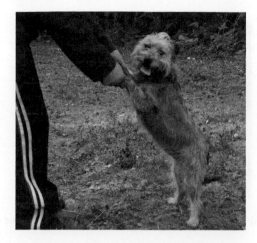

Figure 8.101   *Dancing*. Lift your dog's front legs of the ground and move around for 30 seconds or as long as the dog can stand. Repeat three times twice daily.

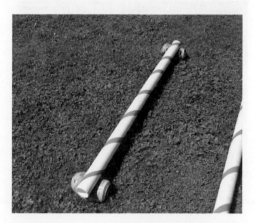

Figure 8.102   *Raised cavaletti poles*. Using crushed cans or blocks to raise poles can make stepping over poles harder and more of a strengthening exercise. Repeat 10 times twice daily.

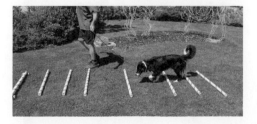

Figure 8.103   *Poles to correct pacing*. Place eight poles in a straight line, measure the height from the floor to the dog's shoulder and use this to measure the distance between the poles. Then as the gait is corrected, take a pole out to encourage the dog to trot correctly for two strides without the poles. Repeat 10 times twice daily.

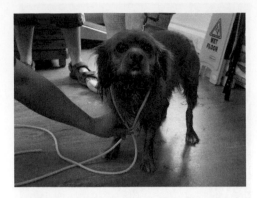

Figure 8.104 *Resistance band to do resisted walking.* Tie a resistance band or tubing around the front of the dog.

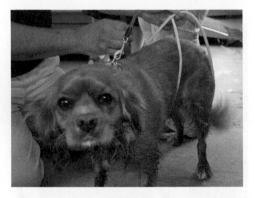

Figure 8.105 *Resistance band to do resisted walking.* Pass the tubing underneath the dog to engage the abdominals.

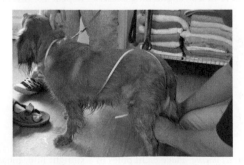

Figure 8.106 *Resistance band to do resisted walking.* Cross the band over the dog's spine and pass over the gluteals to engage them.

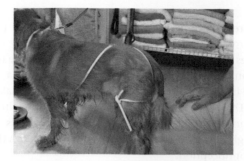

Figure 8.107   *Resistance band to do resisted walking.* Tie the tubing securely, but not too tight on the affected leg. This will give proprioceptive input and strengthen the gluteals and hamstrings as the dog walks. Leave the tubing on for 5 minutes supervised or take the dog for a short walk. Repeat twice daily.

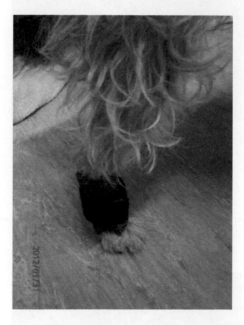

Figure 8.108   *Leg weights.* Place small coins or small sand bags into leg cuffs and place onto the affected leg. Walk the dog for 5–10 minutes twice daily whilst wearing the cuff.

Plyometrics

Advanced muscle strengthening can also be done through the use of plyometrics. Plyometrics is a controlled deceleration followed immediately by a rapid acceleration activity. This activates concentric and eccentric contractions. The theory of plyometrics is that the tension in the muscle fibres is at its greatest after a stretch, and elastic energy will be stored in the elastic elements of the muscle thus making the concentric contraction greater. These exercises must only be used on fit healthy animals and are seen as sport- or work-specific training as they mimic the skills required for these animals, especially agility dogs. They should only be done after a thorough warm up and rely on good proprioception.

Examples of plyometric exercises (Figures 8.109–8.112).

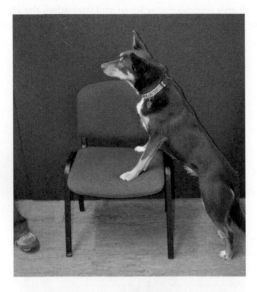

Figure 8.109 *Destination jump.* Ask the dog to jump up onto a chair, bed or into the car. Repeat 10 times twice daily.

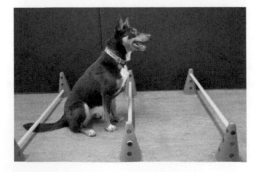

Figure 8.110 *Plyometric jump.* Set a course of jumps, start low and ask the dog to jump over one jump and stop before jumping over the next jump. Repeat the whole course five times twice daily.

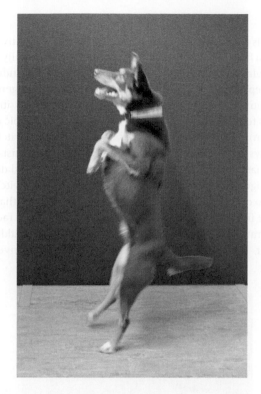

Figure 8.111 *Sit to jump to sit*. Start with the dog sitting and use a treat to encourage it to jump and then sit. Repeat 10 times twice daily.

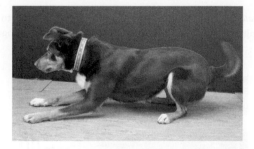

Figure 8.112 *Down to jump to down*. Start with the dog in a down position and use a treat to encourage it to jump up and then go back into the down position. Repeat 10 times twice daily.

Endurance

Muscle endurance is the ability of muscle to perform sustained activity. This can be a singular contraction held over an interval or the ability to continually work at a particular activity. Muscular endurance relies on good cardiovascular endurance or fitness as the ability to keep working will require a good supply of oxygen to the working muscles so the cardiovascular system needs to be as efficient as possible. Muscles have a mix of fibre types to allow them to work in aerobic and anaerobic conditions (with and without oxygen): type I, IIa and IIb fibres. Type I are slow-twitch fibres that rely on aerobic pathways to contract. They are extremely fatigue resistant. Type IIa are fast-twitch fibres that rely on anaerobic pathways to contract and deliver a contraction rapidly but fatigue quickly. Type IIb are intermediate fast-twitch fibres that use aerobic pathways to contract, however are more fatigue resistant than type IIa fibres. The ratio of muscle fibres does rely on genetic disposition, hence racing greyhounds will have a higher ratio of type IIa fibres than a sled dog that would have more type IIb fibres. However, through training, type IIa fibres can be converted to type IIb

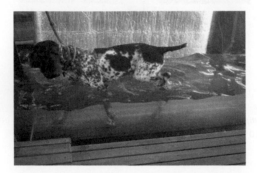

Figure 8.113   *Underwater treadmill.* The underwater treadmill can be used to increase cardiovascular fitness as walking or trotting through resistance will fatigue the dog more quickly than normal walking.

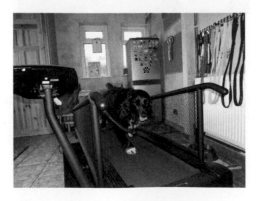

Figure 8.114   Using a treadmill to condition a dog is useful as times, gradient and speed can be carefully monitored.

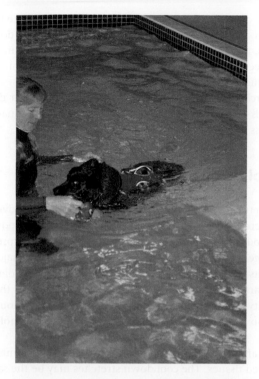

Figure 8.115 Swimming. Swimming can be used to improve cardiovascular fitness, but must be used with caution if the dog has a front leg problem. Swimming for 1 minute is equivalent to walking for 5 minutes.

fibres. Through endurance or resistance training, we can alter the fibre ratio within a muscle and how we do this will depend on the requirements of a dog's performance.

Using an underwater treadmill, normal treadmill and swimming are all good endurance exercises (Figures 8.113–8.115).

Designing a home exercise program

When designing a rehabilitation program, there are many considerations but all programs should address ROM, strength, proprioception and flexibility. The aims/goals of treatment should be discussed with the owner and set together. These goals will form the basis of treatment. If you are treating an agility dog, then towards the end of program they will need to do some sport-specific exercises, such as jumping.

The exercises chosen will depend upon the type of lesion, whether it is being treated surgically or conservatively, tissue affected, stage of healing, current ability of the animal, the capability of the owner to carry out exercises and the prognosis for the animal. A post-operative animal is likely to require passive exercises and static proprioceptive exercises in earlier stages to protect the surgical site. As with all therapeutic interventions, firstly do no harm. Therefore, starting with more basic exercises and progressing the animal, next session may be more appropriate than overloading the lesion too soon and causing further damage. If an exercise does cause pain or increases lameness, then the owner should be advised to stop until it can be seen again and has its technique reassessed. If it is appropriate to continue the exercise, then adapt it or resume with less intensity.

The home exercise program should always be thought as a dynamic process. Reassessment needs to be done regularly to ensure, as the animals improve, they continue to progress towards their final goal.

Warm up/cool down

Clients with dogs returning to sporting activities should also be advised on warm up and cool down exercises that are specific for their dog. The purpose of a warm up is to prepare the body for action, improve the performance and prevent injury. If a dog has no issues, general exercises can be used to activate the major muscle groups to be used during its performance. Warm ups should include cardiovascular activity to increase the heart rate and circulation. Stretches will follow the cardiovascular activity for flexibility and particular attention is paid to any previous areas of injury. A warm up can also be used to ready the dog (and owner) psychologically for their performance.

The cool down after activity is also important to relieve any muscle soreness and stretch any tightened tissues. The cool down stretches may be the same as the warm up stretches. In doing so, the owner may feel whether any changes to the muscles have occurred as a result of activity. This is also important to help the owner recognise when a problem may be beginning and treatment can be sought promptly if required.

The lengths of warm up and cool down will be affected by weather. A cold winter day will require a longer warm up time than a hot summer day, and hence this should be taken into account.

CHAPTER 9
Splints, supports and aids

There are many supports and aids available to enable animals with disabilities and geriatrics to remain functional for a longer time. Casts and splints have been used for several years to immobilise fractured bones and new materials or solutions for these are being developed all the time. Splints, wheels or carts are often used when other options, such as surgery and physiotherapy, have been exhausted or when surgical interventions are not appropriate, for example, a German Shepherd with degenerative myelopathy. We see the use of supports or wraps in sporting dogs to help protect from injury and in animals following surgery or injury to protect the area whilst it heals. There are also numerous companies specialising in making custom orthotics or prosthetics for animals with amputated legs or those with irreversible nerve injuries to enable the animal to remain ambulatory.

When making the decision about which type of device to use, you first need to decide what is the purpose or goal for the device. Does the device need to immobilise a body part or support a joint with pathology? Is it to protect or prevent an injury? Is it being used proactively or to support healing tissues? Is it to correct an existing deformity or to prevent a deformity such as a contracture from occurring? Is it to assist function by supporting weakened muscles or aid sensory loss?

Other considerations that need to be taken into account before choosing a device are the age of the pet that will be wearing the device and whether the device will last for the life expectancy of the pet; the activity level of the animal; what other activities (sporting or working) that the animal might be taking part in and will they be required to be used in challenging environments (outdoors). The size and weight of the pet will influence the appropriateness of certain devices. The owner's ability to take the device on and off, his/her compliance with using the device as instructed and the cost of the device all need to be considered. Finally, the body part being treated needs to be examined for skin integrity, circulation issues and any bony prominences that may cause discomfort for the animal.

Splints

A splint is a rigid device used to support the bones and restrict movement in a certain direction. Traditional splints include aluminium, plastic spoon splints and plaster or fibreglass casts. These are often used for fractures with restricted motion in all directions.

Practical Physiotherapy for Small Animal Practice, First Edition.
Edited by David Prydie and Isobel Hewitt.
© 2015 John Wiley & Sons, Ltd. Published 2015 by John Wiley & Sons, Ltd.
Companion Website: www.wiley.com/go/practical-physiotherapy-for-small-animals

Casts are made to be weight bearing and strong but unlike splints they stay in place and are removed completely rather than be taken on and off as required. This means there is greater potential for pressure sores and soft-tissue injuries in casts. Therefore when using splint and casts, it is extremely important the owner carefully monitors the skin.

Splinting can be used in a wide variety of small animals, although it is most often seen in canine patients. The size variations can make splinting quite challenging, especially in smaller breeds. The use of thermoplastic sheets means splinting is more readily available for veterinarians and therapists to custom-design splints for their clients. Thermoplastic materials are able to fully or partially immobilise a body part as they can withstand high forces and will not crack or break under pressure. The advantages of using thermoplastics for splinting are

The animal does not need to be sedated whilst applying the splint.

The splint is custom made for the animal, improving compliance and reducing the risk of pressure sores.

The body part can be placed into the required position whilst making the splint.

The splint can be modified quickly and easily, if required, at follow-up visits.

It can often be cheaper than other custom-made splints.

Thermoplastic sheets are available in different thicknesses, with or without perforations for airflow around the splint, in different strengths to allow some flexibility around the splint and the differing degrees of conformability (the ease of which the product can be moulded to the patient's body part). These sheets are heated to make them soft and pliable for use. This is done by using hot water. It is important to know how much heat the sheet retains so you are able to work with the material whilst it remains pliable. Once the splint is made, it needs to be cooled to become solid. This process can be speeded up by running cold tap water on it or by wrapping a cold wet crepe bandage over the splint.

Other techniques for splinting are padding, lining and fixing.

Padding materials are used to protect bony prominences, areas of fragile skin and less-protected areas of the body, for example, the tarsus. As Figure 9.1 shows, the padding material affixes directly onto the inside of the splint and can be quite bulky. For this reason, padding should only be used in the middle part of the splint and not end to end as this will significantly alter the fit of the splint particularly with a large amount of padding. The other consideration when using padding is that it can become wet and trap odours, making the splint very unpleasant to wear.

Liners, such as stockinet, can be used instead of padding, but this is much thinner and does not offer as much protection. It has the advantage of being able to be removed and washed, but can more easily move about underneath the splint causing bunching or creasing. This will increase the amount of friction occurring on the skin surface and can cause abrasions. Lining can also be used in the making of splints to cover the whole body part before applying the thermoplastic sheet.

Fixing a splint securely is extremely important for compliance and for the device to be able to carry out its intended use. The two most convenient ways of securing a splint are cohesive wrap and hook and loop straps (VELCRO™). If using cohesive

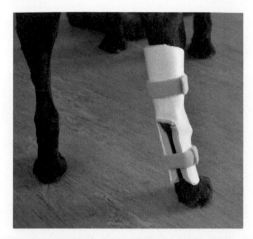

Figure 9.1 *Padding material.* This white tarsal splint with the cut-out piece shows the blue padding material on the inside of the splint to protect the bony prominences around the tarsus.

wrap, consideration needs to be given to the fact that the splint will be held very securely in position, but it will be difficult to monitor the skin surface underneath the wrap. Inspection of the skin will require the wrap to be removed fully and reapplied. Hook and loop straps offer a simple way of enabling owners (and therapists) to apply and remove the splint, allowing them to check the body part regularly. The problem with hook and loop is that it needs to be applied correctly to ensure fixation. If it is too loose, the splint will cause friction and abrasions may occur.

Splinting can be used effectively for Achilles tendinopathies in animals that are not appropriate for surgical management. Figure 9.2 shows a 13-year-old Chocolate Labrador who presented with a swollen and dropped tarsus. She was diagnosed with a

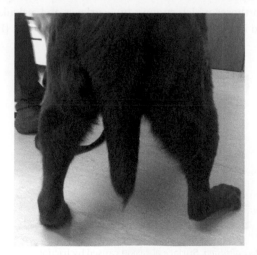

Figure 9.2 *Plantar grade stance.* A 13-year-old Chocolate Labrador diagnosed with a Achilles tendinopathy causing the tarsus to drop into plantigrade stance.

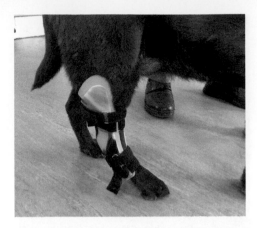

Figure 9.3 *Thermoplastic tarsal splint.* Custom-made thermoplastic splint for an Achilles tendinopathy.

Achilles tendinopathy and the owners decided to manage it conservatively. Figure 9.3 shows the thermoplastic splint made to support the Achilles tendon. Unfortunately, the splint was uncomfortable when worn for long periods and a surface wound developed (Figure 9.4).

Splints can be made for a variety of uses. Legs are most often splinted, but it is possible to make cervical and thoracic collars for support following fractures. Splints are often made by orthotists and occupational therapists in human medicine and there are certain professionals who will also use their specialist skills to make splints for animals. The tarsal splint in Figure 9.3 was made by a human orthotist. If you are unable to find such professionals in your locality, there are companies such as OrthoPets, which can make bespoke splints. They specialise in complex long-term splints that can be bisurfaced orthoses which support two surfaces and articulating braces with hinges incorporated into them to allow for functional movement (Figure 9.5).

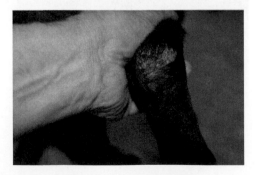

Figure 9.4 *Splint surface abrasion.* Surface abrasion caused by friction between the splint surface and the skin, usually due to a poorly fitting splint.

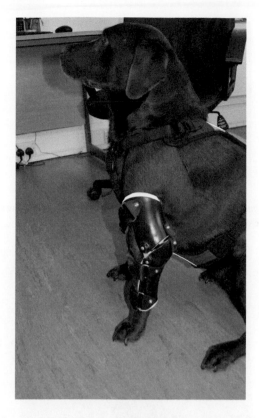

Figure 9.5 *Articulating elbow brace*. This is an example of a custom-made elbow brace for the protection of a total elbow replacement immediately post operation.

Supports

There are a many different supports or wraps available to buy off the shelf for animals. They are usually made from neoprene and have VELCRO™ fastenings to make them adjustable. They will cover the entire body part, provide a thick layer of protection and are easy to clean. Most are for distal leg joints such as the tarsus, carpus, elbow or stifle, although there are some hip and shoulder supports available. Wraps can be used to provide mild to moderate support following grade 1 or 2 ligament strains, to support joints, especially carpus and tarsus, during repetitive activities such as jumping, following fractures if the area is unable to be placed in a cast, for example, scapula and arthritic joints.

Carpal wraps

The amount of support required from a wrap will be directly related to the functional ability of the animal and the stage of its injury or disease. Carpal wraps start with lightweight materials, and light support to be used in sports activities. The level of support can be increased by the addition of additional strengthening. These can be

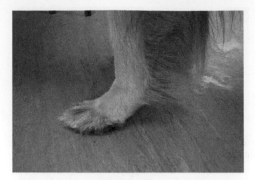

Figure 9.6   *Carpal ligament injury.* The carpus can become dropped following strain to the planter ligaments, causing the dog to adopt a plantigrade stance.

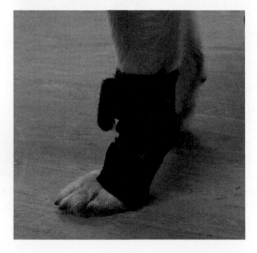

Figure 9.7   *Carpal wrap.* The application of carpal wraps can support the carpus following ligament injury and place the dog back into digitigrade stance to allow normal mobilisation.

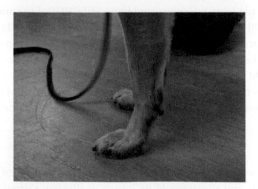

Figure 9.8   *Post carpal wrap.* The same dog in Figure 9.6 following 2 months of wearing the carpal wrap. The wrap prevented possible secondary changes such as contraction of the flexor tendons occurring around the front leg whilst the injury healed.

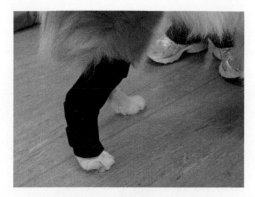

Figure 9.9   *Tarsal wrap.* A neoprene tarsal wrap will provide mild support to the tarsus. This is fixed with hook and loop straps (VELCROTM).

nylon, metallic, wooden or plastic, and for full support, a thermoplastic splint can be added onto the wrap seen in Therapaw's™ carpo-splint kit.

Carpal wraps are designed to stabilise the wrist, prevent hyperextension or protect painful arthritic joints. Figure 9.6 shows a 6-year-old GSD who presented with a front leg lameness and the owner was also complaining of clicking. On observation, it had a hyperextended (dropped) carpus following a ligament strain. It was fitted with a carpal wrap (Figure 9.7). Figure 9.8 shows the carpus after 2 months of wearing the wrap as part of the rehabilitation program.

Tarsal wraps
These are shaped to fit the tarsus comfortably to prevent rubbing around the calcaneus and have varying amounts of support, such as the carpal wraps using nylon straps, plastic or metal inserts. Figure 9.9 shows a tarsal wrap made of neoprene without additional supports and Figure 9.10 shows a tarsal brace with metal medial and lateral supports. This was also used on the 13-year-old Chocolate Labrador Retriever with an Achilles tendinopathy after she was unable to tolerate the thermoplastic splint.

Shoulder braces
The most common shoulder brace used in our clinic is the shoulder stabilisation system from DogLeggs™ or hobbles used for medial shoulder instability. These can also be used for conservative management of MSI, following surgical management of MSI, conservative management of scapular fractures and post-operatively in some shoulder surgeries. The brace has a 'hobble' that prevents abduction of the front legs and it can also limit the amount of flexion and extension at the shoulder whilst still allowing weight bearing. The brace is designed to be worn for long intervals and is generally well tolerated by the animals. A correctly fitting brace is essential. A wide range of sizes is available as is custom fabrication. Owners do not generally have

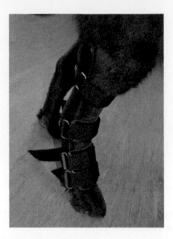

Figure 9.10 *Tarsal brace*. A neoprene tarsal wrap fixed with VELCRO™ straps that provides moderate support due to the addition of medial and lateral metal supports.

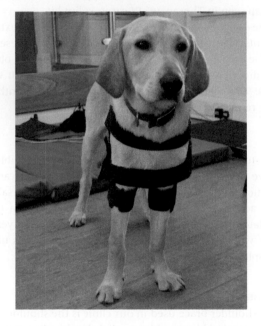

Figure 9.11 *Doggleggs™ shoulder stabilisation system*. This system prevents abduction of the front legs and it can also limit the amount of flexion and extension at the shoulder whilst still allowing weight bearing.

much difficulty applying these and they are usually very compliant with this type of treatment. Figure 9.11 shows an 8-month-old Labrador who slipped and fell whilst playing on a laminate floor and tore the medial joint capsule of the shoulder. This was treated conservatively.

DogLeggs™ also manufacture an elbow brace which is very similar to the shoulder stabilisation system, but does not have the hobble strap. These can be used for protection of the elbow joints in hygroma, ulcers, lick granuloma and arthritic joints.

Hip braces

These can be used for mild hip problems such as dysplasia, pain and arthritis. They are neoprene leggings that cover the upper thigh with a dorsal VELCRO™ fastening which then attaches to a chest harness.

Articulating braces

A range of custom-made articulating braces is available from specialist manufacturers. These can either be set rigid or allow a controlled degree of joint movement. This can be a very useful way of protecting implants and surgeries whilst allowing controlled joint movement. These are available for elbow, carpus, stifle and tarsus (Figure 9.5).

Boots

Boots can be used to protect paws from environmental hazards, such as working dogs in hot deserts, for dogs with proprioceptive deficits to provide more grip or to stop them wearing their claws away.

Dogs with proprioceptive deficits can be helped by using paw grips. These are especially useful if the home environment has wooden floors. Figure 9.12 shows Sticky-Pawz™ that are rubber glove boots. These provide circumferential traction on slippery floors and can be left on during the day.

Tip: The animal's feet can get hot in Sticky-Pawz™. Therefore, use foot powder to prevent moisture build-up or a pin to put few small holes in the boot to create airflow around the foot.

Another type of device to provide traction on slippery floors is Dr. Buzby's™ Toe-Grips (Figure 9.13). These are rubber rings that fit around the dogs nail to provide grip through friction just below the nail tip. Toe grips can also improve proprioceptive input to the paw that can improve gait through increasing awareness of the paw. Dogs tolerate these well. They can be left on as they will wear away naturally, although they should be checked regularly for movement up the nail to the skin of the nail bed.

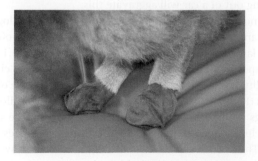

Figure 9.12   *Sticky Pawz™*. These are rubber glove boots that are used to provide circumferential traction on slippery floors in dogs with proprioceptive deficits.

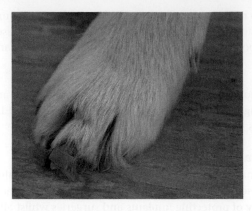

Figure 9.13 *Dr. Buzby's™ ToeGrips*. These are rubber rings that fit around the dog's nail to provide grip through friction just below the nail tip.

Air pressure splints can be applied to legs to help relieve spasticity, prevent contractures and for compression to reduce oedema. They are clear PVC tubes that are placed over the leg and inflated. Once inflated it provides even pressure around the leg.

As with all boots/wraps, it is important to acclimatise the animal to wearing them and if it shows signs of wanting to chew the device, then allow the animal to wear them only under supervision. You can use collars to stop chewing; however, this is likely to distress the animal more.

Aids

Many of our clients have ramps for their dog to get in and out of their car. These are especially useful in the geriatric patients. Ramps offer a solution that helps protect the dog's joints when jumping and the owners back when lifting the dog in and out of the car (Figure 9.14). It is also advisable to have a ramp if the dog has had front-leg surgery, is prone to carpal hyperextension injuries or has a tendency to hyperextend its carpus as jumping out of a car will aggravate this.

Harnesses are another useful aid to help owners to get their dogs mobile. This is particularly important if it is a larger dog to help the owners avoid injuring themselves. There are a large number of harnesses available (Figure 9.15). Animals with cervical injuries, especially following neurosurgery, will require chest harnesses to support their mobility without interfering with the injury site. We often use the Help 'em up™ harnesses (Figures 9.16 and 9.17) as these have two handles. With a number of neurological dogs with back leg involvement the pelvis can be supported, which will significantly help their gait (Figure 9.18). There are also harnesses available with extra long straps. These are useful for small dogs where the owners are likely to damage their back by reaching down to hold the harness.

Another useful adjunct to physiotherapy is the gait retraining aids. These include Dorsi-Flex Assist™ boots and the Biko™ resistance system.

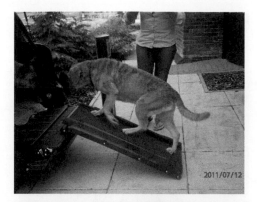

Figure 9.14 *Car ramp.* This offers a solution which helps protect the dog's joints when jumping and the owners back when lifting the dog in and out of the car.

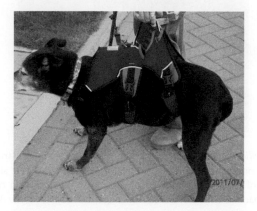

Figure 9.15 *Staffordshire bull terrier wearing a harness.* This was an elderly dog of quite small stature. This type of chest harness was sufficient to support her weight whilst mobilising. It has padded straps and multiple points to adjust the harness for comfort.

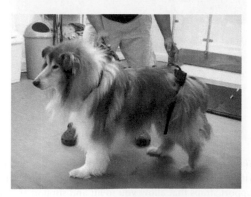

Figure 9.16 *Rough collie in Help 'em up™ harness.* This elderly collie used this harness for 2 years as his mobility decreased. The two handles on chest and hip pad helped to distribute his weight over large surface area, increasing the comfort for the dog and ease of use for the owner.

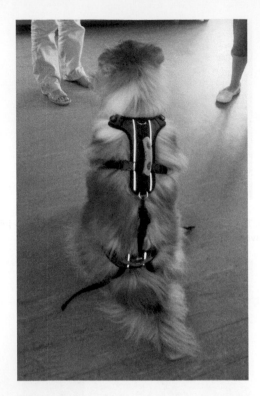

Figure 9.17 *Rough collie in Help 'em up™ harness.* This collie wore the harness all the time as he struggled to walk on slippery surfaces and to step up any inclines or steps. The chest and back pads are made of perforated neoprene to allow the dog to remain cool whilst wearing the harness and are padded with soft fleece, meaning it can be left on the dog for long periods without causing discomfort.

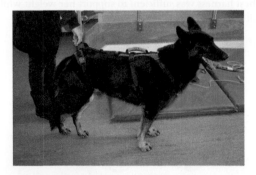

Figure 9.18 *German Shepherd in Help 'em up™ harness.* This dog has degenerative myelopathy and is able to stand with support around the pelvis from the hip lift. The hip lift has a pelvic pad, belly band and support straps that allow you to lift and support the dog's pelvis. This will reduce the strain on the hip joints and the spine.

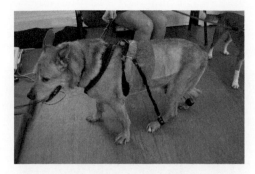

Figure 9.19 *Biko™ progressive resistance bands.* This dog is wearing the Biko™ system which has two leg cuffs that have elastic straps clipped onto them. The elastic straps attach onto a chest harness which is not supplied with the system.

The Biko™ Progressive Resistance Bands is a device that can aid gait where there is bilateral back leg weakness such as degenerative myelopathy, wobblers or degenerative disc disease with mild to moderate ataxia. It consists of two leg cuffs that have elastic straps clipped onto them. These elastic straps attach onto a chest harness. There are different colours of elastic relating to progressive strengths of elastic and it works by pulling the foot forwards as the elastic recoils after being stretched by extending the hips. Caution is needed when selecting clients to use this system on as it does not prevent knuckling and it is not appropriate for acute painful conditions. It is also not suitable for patients with unilateral problems as it can increase ataxia or those with paralysis and no motor function in one or more legs. Figure 9.19 shows a 9-year-old cross breed with a degenerative myelopathy wearing a Biko™ system.

The Dorsi-Flex Assist™ made by Therapaw™ can be used to good effect in dogs and cats that knuckle over on their back legs because of reduced neural input from degenerative myelopathy, peripheral nerve injury or proprioceptive deficits. It can be used in dogs with weakness; however, care needs to be taken to ensure that the dog has enough strength to lift the foot with the boot on and that the dog has enough stability around the hip to control the movement of the leg. The elastic straps are placed under tension and as the animal brings the leg forwards, the elastic aids the foot being moved up into dorsiflexion. Figure 9.20 shows a back leg Dorsi-Flex Assist™. It is also available for the front leg, again stability is required at the shoulder to use this.

In our clinic, we also see a large number of dogs with degenerative myelopathies. These can be fairly active dogs whose neurological deficit is reducing their activity levels. In these cases, carts can give these dogs a new lease of life. Figure 9.21 shows a 10-year-old German Shepherd, who initially presented at our clinic with weakness and lameness of her back legs which were reducing her mobility over 2 years. The treatment she received included acupuncture and hydrotherapy, but she was unable to stand unassisted. The set of wheels has increased her activity levels and, improved her quality of life enormously again. Figure 9.22 shows a 13-year-old Border Collie

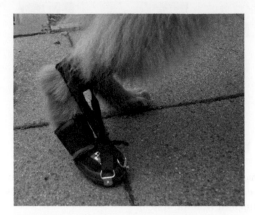

Figure 9.20   *Dorsi-Flex Assist™.* This dog is wearing the back leg Dorsi-Flex Assist™. It consists of a boot, elastic straps and the leg cuff. The elastic straps are placed under tension and as the animal brings the leg forwards, the elastic aids the foot being moved up into dorsiflexion.

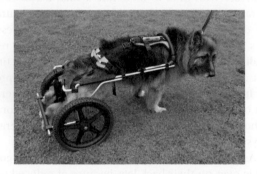

Figure 9.21   *German Shepherd in a cart.* The dog is in a cart made by Eddie's Wheels and enables her to stand and mobilise unassisted by supporting her back legs.

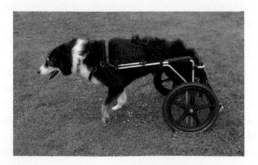

Figure 9.22   *Border Collie in a cart.* This dog is able to mobilise in his wheelchair despite having severe muscle wasting of his back legs due to degenerative myelopathy. This type of cart is very light but very strong.

with degenerative myelopathy who presented at our clinic with a 3-year history of reduced mobility and weakness of his back legs. Before using the wheels, he was unable to stand unaided because of the severe muscle wasting in his back legs. The two different types of wheels shown are not the only ones available and selection of the most appropriate ones for your client should be done on an individual basis. There are certain criteria that should be met for all dogs; they should be fully adjustable; able to be used on a variety of surfaces and of sturdy construction.

CHAPTER 10
Pain

This chapter will aim to identify the signs of pain in dogs and cats as well as the management of that pain from a practical point of view in practice. This chapter will only touch on the neurophysiology of pain. For more details on this, please see further reading.

Pain can be divided into acute and chronic. Acute pain is a defence mechanism that helps prevent further injury or damage to an area that has already suffered insult. However, to withhold analgesia in order to prevent movement of a post operative patient is unacceptable. Chronic or maladapted pain has no physiological function.

Signs of pain

Because animals cannot communicate verbally, signs of pain are behavioural and emotional. Various schemes have been developed for the assessment of pain in practice (Glasgow Composite Measure Pain Scale – CMPS – SF, University of Melbourne Pain Score – UMPS and University of Colorado Canine Chronic Pain Scale). All of these schemes give a score for various parameters. This score can then be monitored for improvement or worsening of pain. The authors would encourage every practice to use these forms. Links to the websites to download these forms are given in Appendix 3, Useful Websites.

Signs of pain in the dog may include decreased appetite, depressed unresponsive behaviour, hiding at the back of the kennel, reluctance to stand or walk, indifference when shown a lead, whimpering or vocalisation, licking at a specific area and drooling.

Signs to look for in a cat may include lack of grooming, drooling, hiding at the back of the kennel, dilated pupils, vocalisation, growling, hissing and aggression when approached.

Physiology of pain

Pain in a joint will be used to describe the basic neurophysiology of pain.

Practical Physiotherapy for Small Animal Practice, First Edition.
Edited by David Prydie and Isobel Hewitt.
© 2015 John Wiley & Sons, Ltd. Published 2015 by John Wiley & Sons, Ltd.
Companion Website: www.wiley.com/go/practical-physiotherapy-for-small-animals

Innervation

A joint has the following neuroreceptors: mechanoreceptors, nociceptors and silent nociceptors.

Mechanoreceptors

These respond to mechanical stimuli such as tension and pressure, and are activated by joint movement. They send information rapidly to the CNS about the spacial awareness and orientation of the joint and leg.

Nociceptors

These detect stimuli that actually or potentially could cause tissue damage. They are divided into subtypes according to the fibre type.

Aα fibres are large myelinated fibres that allow rapid transmission to the spinal cord. They are present in ligaments. They respond to potentially damaging mechanical stimuli.

Aδ fibres respond to mechanical, thermal and chemical stimuli. They are myelinated but of smaller diameter than Aα fibres. They are found throughout the joint and subchondral bone with the exception of the cartilage which is aneural and avascular.

C fibres respond to similar stimuli as Aδ fibres, but are of small diameter and are unmyelinated. The distribution of C fibres is the same as Aδ.

Silent nociceptors are present but inactive in normal joints. However, when inflammation is present they become sensitised.

Mechanoreceptor and nociceptor fibres run to the dorsal horn of the spinal cord where they synapse. They can form a local arc back to the periarticular muscles causing muscle contraction. Impulses also ascend the spinal cord to the brain. These signals are subject to ascending and descending modulations (Figure 10.1).

When cell injury occurs, the arachidonic acid cascade (Figure 10.4) results in the formation of inflammatory mediators that stimulate the nociceptors, resulting in pain.

Local sensitisation

If the pain goes unchecked, local sensitisation can occur. There is a build-up of inflammatory mediators that lower the threshold response of the Aδ and C fibre nociceptors. A mild nociceptive input will produce an exaggerated pain response that may last for some time. The area becomes hyperalgesic (Figure 10.2).

Central sensitisation

In this situation, nerve fibres that are not usually associated with nociception also become recruited in pain transmission. This results in actions such as stroking that would not normally produce pain to result in pain. This is known as allodynia. In this situation, changes take place in the dorsal horn, spinal cord and brain that amplify the sensation of pain (Figure 10.3).

Management of pain

Pain is best managed using a multimodal approach. This may be achieved by using a combination of drugs and other techniques that act in different ways.

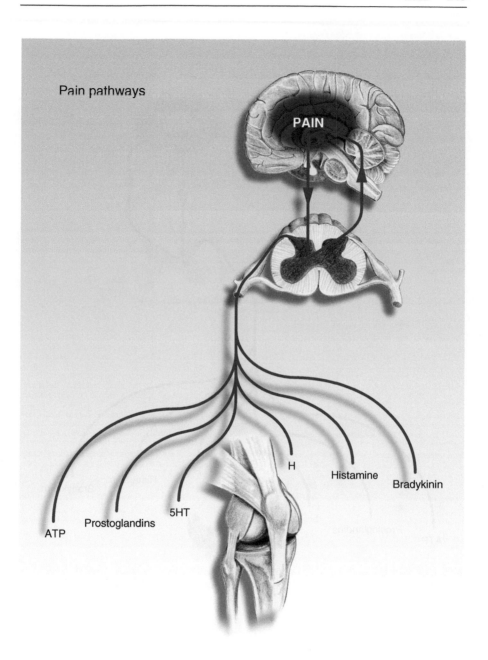

Figure 10.1   Normal neurotransmission from around a joint.

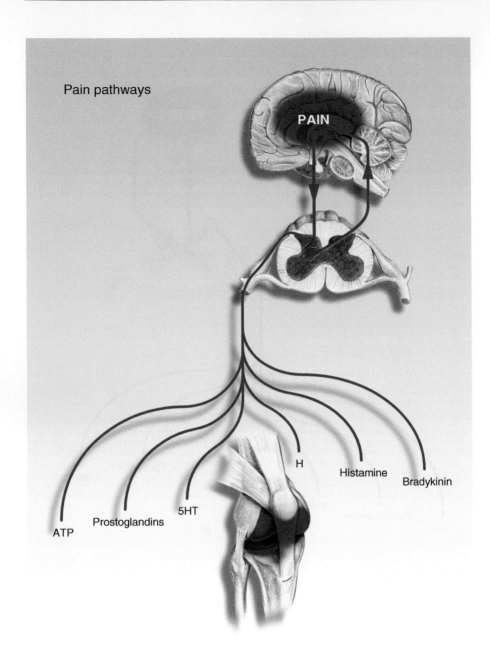

Figure 10.2 *Local sensitisation.* Hyperaesthesia results in an area of higher than expected pain response to a painful stimulus.

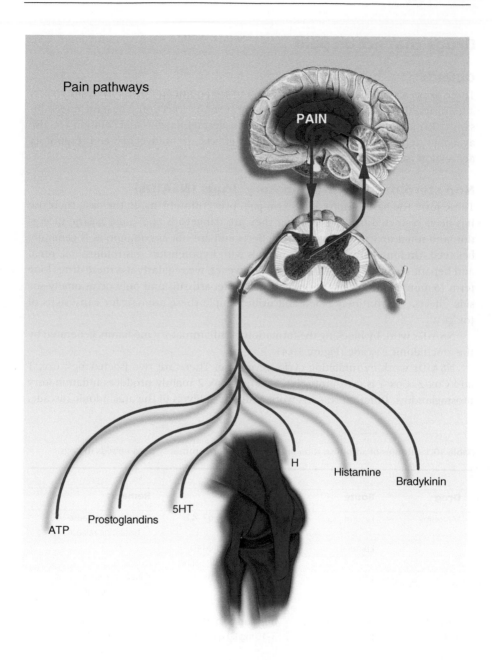

Figure 10.3 *Central sensitisation (Allodynia)*. Neurons which would normally transmit proprioception and mechanical information now transmit pain.

Drugs that act on pain

Opioids

These drugs act centrally and peripherally and are potent analgesics. They are mostly administered perioperatively usually by intravenous injection, constant rate infusion (CRI) and/or via the epidural route. Transdermal patches and solution are also available (fentanyl). The most common side effects are bradycardia and respiratory depression (see Tables 10.1 and 10.2).

Non-steroidal anti-inflammatory drugs (NSAIDs)

These form the basis of most long-term pain prevention plans. In the past, their use has been restricted in the belief that they are dangerous and cause gastric ulceration and renal toxicity. These are side effects and are not as common as is generally believed. Undoubtedly their use in animals with hypotension, gastrointestinal, renal and hepatic disorders should be avoided. However, we regularly use these drugs long term (6 months to 8 years) in animals with osteoarthritis and only occasionally see side effects. We routinely blood and urine sample these animals for early signs of toxicity.

NSAIDs work by blocking the formation of inflammatory mediators generated by the arachidonic cascade (Figure 10.4).

NSAIDs work by inhibiting cyclo-oxygenase. There are two isoenzymes: Cox 1 and Cox 2. Cox 1 is cyto-protective, whereas Cox 2 mainly produces inflammatory prostaglandins. Different NSAIDs work at different levels of the arachidonic cascade.

Table 10.1   Routes of administration and dose rates for commonly used opioids in dogs.

		Dogs	
Drug	**Route**	**Dose**	**Remarks**
Morphine	I.v., i.m., s.c.	0.2–0.5 mg/kg q3–4 h	Rapid i.v. can cause histamine release
	Epidural	0.1 mg/kg diluted to 0.2 ml/kg with saline	
	CRI	0.1–0.2 mg/kg/h	Can be mixed with ketamine and lignocaine
Methadone	Slow i.v., i.m., s.c.	0.1–0.6 mg/kg q4 h	Apnoea when given i.v.
Pethidine	I.m., s.c.	3–10 mg/kg q1–2 h	Do not give intravenously as it causes massive histamine release
Fentanyl	I.v.	1–5 µg/kg q 30 min	
	CRI	Loading dose 1–2 µg/kg followed by 0.05–0.15 µg/kg/h	
	Transdermal	4 µg/kg/h	
Buprenorphine	I.v., i.m.	0.01–0.02 mg/kg q6–8 h	Can use on oral mucosa at 0.12 mg/kg
Butorphanol	I.v., i.m.	0.2–0.4 mg/kg q2 h	

Table 10.2   Opioids commonly used in cats.

Drug	Route	Dose	Remarks
		Cats	
Morphine	I.v., i.m., s.c.	0.1–0.4 mg/kg q3–4 h	Rapid i.v. can cause histamine release
	Epidural	0.1 mg/kg diluted to 0.2 ml/kg with saline	
Methadone	Slow i.v., i.m., s.c.	0.1–0.3 mg/kg q4 h	Apnoea when given i.v.
Pethidine	I.m., s.c.	5–10 mg/kg q1–2 h	Do not give intravenously as it causes massive histamine release
Fentanyl	I.v.	2–5 µg/kg q30 min	
	CRI	Loading dose 1–2 µg/kg followed by 0.05–0.15 µg/kg/h	
	Transdermal	25 µg/kg/h	
Buprenorphine	I.v., i.m.	0.01–0.02 mg/kg q6–8 h	Can use on oral mucosa at 0.12 mg/kg
Butorphanol	I.v., i.m.	0.1–0.4 mg/kg q2 h	

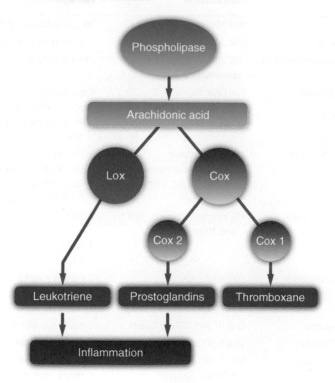

Arachidonic acid cascade

Figure 10.4   The Arachidonic Cascade starts in response to phospholipids released from the damaged cell membrane.

Diets rich in Omega 3 EPA (eicosapentaenoic acid) also affect the arachidonic cascade and reduce pain. The EPA replaces some of the arachidonic acid. This has the effect of dampening down the cascade.

Aspirin has no Cox specificity. Phenylbutazone, cincophen (part of prednoleucotropin – PLT tablets) and ketoprofen are Cox 1 selective. Carprofen (Rimadyl) and meloxicam (Metacam) are Cox 2 selective. The newer coxib NSAID drugs, robenacoxib (Onsior), firocoxib (Previcox) and cimicoxib (Cimalgex) are Cox 2 specific. Also the action of mavacoxib (Trocoxil) lasts for 28 days from a single oral dose (see below). Tables 10.3 and 10.4 show the commonly used NSAIDs in small-animal practice and their dose rate.

Toxicity issues of NSAIDs

Some dogs will be NSAID intolerant. Some dogs show signs immediately, whereas others may not show signs until they have been on NSAIDs for some time. NSAIDs can cause intestinal irritation and ulceration. They can also adversely affect the kidneys and liver.

Clinical signs of toxicity may vary, but can include loss of appetite, drooling, signs of abdominal pain, vomiting, which may contain 'coffee grounds', diarrhoea,

Table 10.3 Common NSAIDs used in dogs.

Drug	Formulation	Dosage
Aspirin	Oral 75 and 300 mg tablets	10–20 mg/kg p.o. q12 h
Phenylbutazone	Oral 100 and 200 mg tablets	2–20 mg/kg p.o. 8–12 h
Cinchofen/prednisolone (PLT)	Oral 200 mg tablets + 1 mg prednisolone	25 mg/kg q12 h
Cartrophen (Rimadyl)	Injectable 50 mg/ml. Oral 20, 50 and 100 mg tablets	4 mg/kg i.v., s.c. 4 mg/kg q24 h orally as loading dose dropping to 2 mg/kg q24 h
Meloxicam (Metacam)	2 mg/ml injectable 1.5 mg/ml oral suspension. Oral 1.0 and 2.5 mg tablets	0.2 mg/kg s.c. 0.2 mg/kg p.o. as a single loading dose followed by 0.1 mg/kg p.o.q24 h
Ketoprofen (Ketophen)	1% injectable solution. Oral 5 and 20 mg tablets	2 mg/kg i.v., i.m., s.c. q24 up to 3 days 1 mg/kg p.o. q24 h for up to 5 days
Robenacoxib (Onsior)	20 mg/ml solution Oral 5, 10, 20 and 40 mg tablets	2 mg/kg s.c. q24 h for up to 2 days 1 mg/kg p.o. q24 h
Firocoxib (Previcox)	Oral 57 and 227 mg tablets	5 mg/kg p.o. q24 h
Cimicoxib (Cimalgex)	Oral 8, 30 and 80 mg tablets	2 mg/kg p.o. q24 h
Mavacoxib (Trocoxil)	Oral 6, 20, 30, 75 and 95 mg tablets	2 mg/kg p.o. q14 d for two doses. Then q 28 d for a total of seven doses

Table 10.4   Common NSIADS used in cats.

Drug	Formulation	Dosage
Cartrophen (Rimadyl)	Injectable 50 mg/ml	4 mg/kg i v , s.c. single dose
Meloxicam (metacam)	2 mg/ml injectable Oral 0.5 mg/ml oral suspension	0.2 mg/kg s.c. single injection 0.1 mg/kg p.o. as a single loading dose followed by 0.05 mg/kg p.o. q24 h
Ketoprofen (Ketofen)	1% injectable solution. Oral 5 and 20 mg tablets	2 mg/kg i.v., i.m., s.c. q24 up to 3 days 1 mg/kg p.o. q24 h for up to 5 days
Robenacoxib (Onsior)	20 mg/ml solution Oral 6 mg tablets	2 mg/kg s.c. q24 h for up to 2 days 1–2 mg/kg p.o. q24 h for up to 6 days

melaena, polydypsia, polyuria and anaemia. Animals on long-term NSAIDs should have routine blood work. If signs of toxicity appear, the NSAIDs should be stopped immediately. Another form of pain relief should be given. Mild gastric irritation may respond to cimetidine (dogs 5–10 mg/kg q8 h, cats 2.5–5 mg/kg q8 h) or ranitidine (dogs 2 mg/kg q8–12 h, cats 3.5 mg/kg q12 h), but ulceration will require omeprazole (dogs 0.5–1.5 mg/kg i.v., p.o. q24, cats 0.75–1 mg/kg p.o. q24 h). Animals with signs of renal or hepatic issues will need fluid therapy and renal/hepatic support.

Other drugs used in managing pain.

Ketamine

Given at sub-anaesthetic doses this is thought to have strong analgesic properties especially when used as part of a continuous rate infusion with other drugs, such as morphine and lignocaine.

Local anaesthetic

These agents can be used to create a regional block. They are also regularly used as part of a continuous rate infusion in acute pain.

Alpha-2 agonists

These drugs are being used more and more to treat acute pain. They also have the advantage of sedation. This reduces anxiety, that is, a major contributing factor to pain in humans.

Paracetamol (Acetaminophen)

This drug is useful as an adjunct to NSAIDs in the management of OA pain. It is also useful in NSAID-intolerant dogs. If given long term, regular blood work is essential to monitor hepatic function. The mode of action is unclear, but we regularly use it in combination with NSAIDs with few problems.

Tramadol

It has become popular recently for treating pain in dogs. In our hands, the effect seems very variable with many patients showing no reduction in pain levels. It does seem to cause drowsiness in a significant number of dogs. The recommended dosage is high compared to the dose in man.

Gabapentin

It was originally introduced as an anticonvulsant drug, but is now used more commonly to treat chronic pain, especially if central sensitisation is present.

Amantadine

It is an antiviral drug, but appears to enhance the pain relief of other drugs such as NSAIDs when given in combination (see Tables 10.5 and 10.6).

Selection of medication in chronic pain

Often the selection of NSAIDs or other analgesic medication is arrived at randomly by the veterinary surgeon. If the first-choice medication is unsuccessful, there is often no logical plan to finding an effective regime. As an example of this, we will use the case of the chronic OA patient and describe how we work through the drugs in a logical manner. At first presentation, an NSAID would be prescribed unless there was a history of NSAID intolerance, renal or hepatic disease. The dog would then be checked 1 week later. If clinical signs had improved, the NSAIDs would be continued and the dog seen in 3-4 weeks. If there had been no improvement, the first NSAID would be stopped and replaced by another NSAID allowing a washout period. The dog would again be seen in 7 days.

In the first case where the dog had improved, if there had been no further lameness, the dog would be signed off for 3 months. If the dog had gone lame again, it would be put back onto NSAID 1 for 1 month and re-seen after that period.

In the second case that had been put onto NSAID 2, if there had been improvement, the dog would be left on that NSAID for a further month and re-examined at that time. If there had been little or no improvement in clinical signs, a first adjunct would be added. My (DP) first choice is paracetamol (acetaminophen). The dog would be seen in a further 7 days. If there had been improvement in clinical signs, the NSAID 2/paracetamol (acetaminophen) would be continued for a further 7 days. The paracetamol (acetaminophen) would then be stopped but continued on NSAID 2 for a further 14 days when the dog would be re-examined. If there had still been no improvement, a second adjunct, tramadol, would be added and the dog re-examined in 7 days. If after 7 days there were still no improvement, gabapentin or amantadine would be added to the mix. Once pain has been controlled, which may take several weeks or months, the adjuncts would be withdrawn. If the dog was still showing pain when on NSAIDs, paracetamol (acetaminophen), tramadol and gabapentin, the diagnosis would be reconsidered as would the quality of life. We would also use a multimodal approach to the OA case (Chapter 11). As stated earlier, we tend to leave the chronic OA dogs on NSAIDs for several months before considering withdrawal.

Table 10.5 Other drugs used to treat pain in dogs.

Drug	Route	Dogs	
		Dosage	Remarks
Ketamine	CRI	Loading dose 0.5 mg/kg followed by CRI of 5 µg/kg/min	Maximum 24–36 h
Lignocaine	Perineural	2–4 mg/kg	Duration 1 h
Bupivacaine	CRI	Loading dose 1–1.5 mg/kg followed by CRI of 50 µg/kg/min	
	Perineural	1–1.5 mg/kg	Duration 4–6 h. *DO NOT GIVE INTRAVENOUSLY*
Medetomidine	I.v., i.m.	1–2 µg/kg	Synergistic action with opioids. Bradycardia
	CRI	1–2 µg/kg/h	
Dexmedetomidine	I.v., i.m.	0.5–1 µg/kg	
	CRI	0.5–1 µg/kg/h	
Paracetamol (acetaminophen) 400 mg combined with 9 mg of codeine (pardale V)	Oral 400 + 9 mg codeine tablet 500 mg tablet	10 mg/kg q 12 h	*DO NOT USE IN CATS*
Tramadol	Oral 50, 100, 200 and 300 mg slow-release tablets	5 mg/kg q 8 h	Do not use with tricyclic antidepressants or monoamine oxidase inhibitors
Gabapentin	Oral 100, 300 and 400 capsules 600 and 800 mg tablets	10–60 mg/kg	Incremental dosing recommended
Amantadine (lysovir)	Oral 100 mg capsule: 10 mg/ml syrup	3–5 mg mg/kg q24 h	

Table 10.6   Other drugs used to treat pain in cats.

		Cats	
Drug	**Route**	**Dosage**	**Remarks**
Ketamine	CRI	Loading dose 0.5 mg/kg followed by CRI of 5 µg/kg/min	Maximum 24–36 h
Lignocaine	Perineural	2–4 mg/kg	Duration 1 h
	CRI	Loading dose 1–1.5 mg/kg followed by CRI of 50 µg/kg/min	
Bupivacaine	Perineural	1–1.5 mg/kg	Duration 4–6 h. *DO NOT GIVE INTRAVENOUSLY*
Medetomidine	I.v., i.m.	1–2 µg/kg	Synergistic action with opioids. Bradycardia
	CRI	1–2 µg/kg/h	
Dexmedetomidine	I.v., i.m.	0.5–1 µg/kg	
	CRI	0.5–1 µg/kg/h	
Tramadol	Oral 50, 100, 200 and 300 mg slow-release tablets	2–4 mg/kg q 8 h	Do not use with tricyclic antidepressants or monoamine oxidase inhibitors
Gabapentin	Oral 100, 300 and 400 mg capsules 600 and 800 mg tablets	5–10 mg/kg	Incremental dosing recommended
Amantadine (lysovir)	Oral 100 mg capsule: 10 mg/ml syrup	1–4 mg mg/kg q24 h	Incremental dosing recommended

Other practices affecting pain

Modalities (see Chapter 4)

Some modalities also produce pain relief. The use of ice immediately post operation or post injury can significantly reduce pain. It does so by reducing cell metabolism in the area of damage and reducing inflammation. The application of cold also slows down both sensory and motor nerve conduction velocities.

While cooling is of use in treating acute pain, heat can be used as an adjunct in chronic pain.

Massage

This will increase blood supply to an area and is useful at relieving muscle tension and myofascial trigger points.

TENS

This can be used to numb pain between the electrical pads. The pain relief, however, will only be effective whilst the current is flowing.

LASER

In addition to increasing blood supply to an area, lasers also cause the release of endorphins that can have a profound effect on pain.

PEMFT

Pulsed electromagnetic field therapy (PEMFT) is thought to interfere with nerve transmission in small unmyelinated nerves such as C fibres. We certainly observe behavioural changes in cats that we treat with PEMFT. They go from being hidden at the back of the carrier curled up as small as possible and hissing when approached to relaxed sleeping cats which allow stroking. All we do is place the carrier on the PEMFT mat and switch on for 20 minutes.

Hydrotherapy

We use hydrotherapy a lot in the management of our chronic OA patients. Often we will place the patient in the UWTM and fill to mid femur with warm water. Sometimes we do not start the conveyor belt but just let the dogs stand in the warm water for 15 minutes. The theory is that the hydrostatic pressure exerted by the water on the body of the patient will help reduce the venous congestion in the sub-chondral bone, thought to be a major cause of pain in OA sufferers.

Surgery

This can have a dramatic effect in certain situations. A good example would be a total hip replacement for chronic painful hip arthritis. Another example would be attenuation of pain following amputation for osteosarcoma.

Acupuncture

A full explanation of how acupuncture works is beyond the scope of this textbook. A brief description of the 'Western' explanation will be given.

Acupuncture involves the inserting of fine needles into a patient (Figure 10.5). In animals, this is considered an act of veterinary medicine and can only be carried out by a qualified veterinary surgeon. It is possible to stimulate acupuncture points using a laser or pressure. These procedures are not true acupuncture.

Acupuncture to treat pain

Acupuncture requires an intact nervous system. Local anaesthetic will block the effect of acupuncture. Acupuncture is in part mediated by endorphins and other opiates. Giving opiate antagonists will stop acupuncture from working. Acupuncture is thought to upregulate messenger RNA so as to produce more opiates at subsequent treatments.

When acupuncture needles are inserted into the skin, they stimulate the myelinated Aδ fibres. These fibres signal potential tissue damage and withdraw the body from the threatening stimulus. In doing so, the brain and dorsal horn override the chronic pain being transmitted by the unmyelinated C fibres.

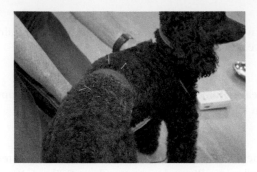

Figure 10.5   Dog undergoing acupuncture for chronic neck pain.

After having its effect at the dorsal horn, acupuncture stimulus travels via the spinal cord to the brain. This triggers release of endorphins and other neurotransmitters that have a pain-relieving modulation on the descending pathways.

Acupuncture is also very useful for treating myofascial trigger points. These regularly occur in the paraspinal muscles and direct needling of these points brings effective pain relief.

CHAPTER 11

Treatment protocols

In this chapter, we try to give guidance to possible treatment plans for specific conditions. However, please be aware that these are just general guidelines. Every case is different and will require a *Subjective* (history), *Objective* (clinical findings), *Analysis* and identification of problems and drawing up of an individual *Plan* (*SOAP*). The plan will change as the patient progresses through the recovery phases, and hence frequent reviews are vital.

Shoulder

Osteochondritis dissecans (OCD)

Signalment. Usually immature growing dog, often large breed with foreleg lameness. Poor response to NSAIDS. Pain on shoulder flexion and extension. May have atrophy of supraspinatus muscle.

Diagnosis. X-ray, arthroscopy and MRI (Figure 11.1).

Treatment. Most will be treated by surgical removal of the cartilage flap either by open surgery or by arthroscopy. Severe cases may have had a cartilage core graft.

Post–operative Rehabilitation.

Days 1–5

    Focus for management. Surgical wound, swelling and post-operative pain management. Minimise muscle loss.

    Pain relief. Opiates/NSAIDS as appropriate.

    Environment. Check for suitable flooring and have the owner put down rugs and runners as required.

    Diet. Weight loss as required. Consider inclusion of EPA in diet.

    Exercise. Lead walk on level even ground for 2 minutes twice daily. No stairs, games or playing with other dogs.

    Modalities. Apply ice to the wound for 10 minutes twice daily. Laser at $2\,j/cm^2$ at joint surface every other day.

    Pulsed electromagnetic field therapy every other day set for pain relief (see manufacturers' instructions).

    Electrical muscle stimulation (EMS) to supraspinatus and spinous head of deltoid for 10 minutes twice weekly.

Practical Physiotherapy for Small Animal Practice, First Edition.
Edited by David Prydie and Isobel Hewitt.
© 2015 John Wiley & Sons, Ltd. Published 2015 by John Wiley & Sons, Ltd.
Companion Website: www.wiley.com/go/practical-physiotherapy-for-small-animals

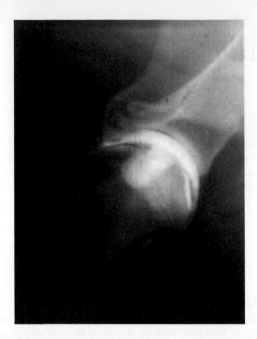

Figure 11.1 Contrast arthrogram of the left shoulder showing OCD flap.

Therapeutic exercise. Passive range of motion. Flex and extend the joint in the midrange. Hold in flexion and extension for 15 seconds each. Three repetitions repeated twice daily (Fig. 8.2 and Fig. 8.3).

Days 6–14

Focus for management. Range of motion, proprioception and core stability.

Pain relief. NSAIDS.

Exercise. Lead walk 5 minutes twice daily. No stairs, games or playing with other dogs.

Modalities. Continue laser, PEMFT and EMS twice weekly.

Therapeutic exercise. Continue PROM exercises as per days 1–5. Introduce Cream cheese to the axilla (Fig. 8.37) three times twice daily. Introduce Biscuits from the Shoulders, Ribs and Hips (Figs. 8.27–29). Five repetitions of each twice daily.

Days 14–30

Focus for management. Muscle building.

Pain relief. NSAIDS as required.

Exercise. Lead walk 10 minutes twice daily. No stairs, games or playing with other dogs.

Modalities. Continue laser and PEMFT weekly. Introduce hydrotherapy either in UWTM with water just above feet to encourage AROM for 4 minutes gradually building up to 8 minutes or in the pool doing therapeutic exercises on platforms. Introduce assisted swimming.

Therapeutic exercise. Continue Biscuits from Shoulder, Ribs and Hips as per days 6–14, but increase repetitions to 10 repetitions twice daily. Introduce High Five (Fig. 8.35) and Down to Sit (Fig. 8.33–34) five repetitions twice daily. Also introduce Cavaletti Pole work (Fig. 8.77) – five passes twice daily.

Days 31–90

Focus for management. Muscle Strengthening.

Pain relief. NSAIDS as required.

Exercise. Twice daily 20 minutes on lead. Introduce gentle inclines and declines. The dog can be allowed off lead for 5 minutes twice daily. Dog is allowed to go up and down stairs twice daily. No games or playing with other dogs.

Modalities. UWTM/pool weekly building up to 20 minutes per session. Increase depth of water to cover elbow if using UWTM. Introduce free swimming if using pool.

Therapeutic exercise. Continue High five and Down to Sit, but increase to 10 repetitions twice daily. Add Side Stepping (Fig. 8.95) 3 m (10 ft) in both directions repeated three times twice daily.

Days 91–120

Focus for management. Muscle strengthening and return to normal activity.

Exercise. Twice daily 45–60 minutes twice daily on lead. The dog can be allowed off lead for 15 minutes twice daily. Games or playing with other dogs for 5 minutes.

Modalities. Continue hydrotherapy as for days 31–90. Consider introducing land treadmill.

Therapeutic exercise. Continue for days 31–90, but introduce a third repetition.

Shoulder tendinopathies

These conditions usually have an insidious onset and can occur together or individually. They are often present in medial shoulder instability (see later).

Supraspinatus tendinopathy

In this condition, calcification occurs in the tendon of insertion of the supraspinatus muscle. Occasionally, the calcification can be a discreet entity that can be surgically removed but in most cases the calcification is diffuse. The tendon runs close to the tendon of origin of the biceps brachii and can impinge on the biceps through the joint capsule.

Signalment. These dogs usually present with a varying degree of foreleg lameness with an insidious onset. Response to NSAIDS is poor. The lameness is often worse after exercise. The supraspinatus muscle belly is atrophied. There is pain on digital pressure directly on the tendon. Many of these dogs will have a positive biceps stress test. Shoulder flexion is often reduced.

Diagnosis. X-ray, arthroscopy, diagnostic ultrasound and MRI (Figure 11.2).

Treatment. Modalities and therapeutic exercise.

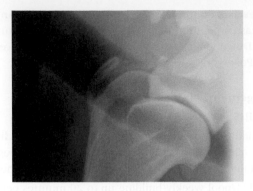

Figure 11.2   Radiograph of a shoulder showing calcified nodules in the tendon of supraspinatus.

Days 1–7

Focus for management. Restarting the inflammatory process. Often the process of inflammation has ceased before healing is complete. Restarting the inflammation will bring new blood vessels that will enhance repair. For this reason, NSAIDS and other anti-inflammatory drugs should be avoided.

   The installation of platelet-rich plasma or stem cells into the tendon should also be considered as part of the treatment plan.

Pain relief. Acetaminophen (paracetamol), tramadol

Environment. Advise no stairs, check for slippery flooring. Advise lift in and out of car or use a ramp.

Exercise. Twice daily 10 minutes on lead on flat even ground. No ball games or playing with other dogs.

Day 1

Modalities. Shockwave. 600–2000 shocks depending on type of shockwave and patient weight delivered over the tendons and muscle bellies of supraspinatus and biceps brachii. Shockwave not only kick-starts the inflammatory process, but acts to break up the areas of calcification.

If shock wave is not available, then treat with laser (12 j/cm^2 at target tissue, Chapter 5) daily over the same area. Pulsed ultrasound (3.3 MHz, 20%, 2.0 W/cm^2, Chapter 5) for 5 minutes twice weekly. PEMFT twice weekly on settings to encourage vascularisation (see manufacturers' instructions).

Manual therapies. Cross-frictional massage (Chapter 6) to the tendon for 2 minutes twice daily in an attempt to stimulate inflammatory response.

Therapeutic exercise. Passive Shoulder ROM and stretching of supraspinatus and biceps muscles, three repetitions twice daily (Figs. 8.2–3, 8.49).

Days 8–14

Focus for management. Management of inflammatory response. Maintaining ROM. Start of early strengthening exercises.

Exercise. Increase lead exercise to 15 minutes twice daily on level even ground. No games or playing with other dogs.

Modalities. Laser twice weekly and pulsed ultrasound twice weekly *OR* repeat shockwave on day 14. PEMFT twice weekly.

Therapeutic exercise. Increase stretches to five repetitions twice daily. Introduce active ROM by using Cavaletti Pole work (Fig. 8.77) 10 reps twice daily, 3 repetitions twice daily. Introduce strengthening exercises High Five 5 repetitions twice daily (Fig. 8.35) and Down to a Sit (Fig. 8.33–34) 5 repetitions twice daily.

Days 15–28

Focus for management. ROM and strengthening.

Exercise. Twice daily 20 minutes twice daily on lead on level even ground. No games or playing with other dogs.

Modalities. Laser and ultrasound weekly *OR* shockwave day 28. PEMFT twice weekly. Introduce hydrotherapy twice weekly. Walking in the UWTM with water just below shoulder height for 2 minutes. If in pool, do High Five (Fig. 8.35) exercises and Three Leg Standing (Fig. 8.61). Caution with swimming.

Therapeutic exercise. Five stretches twice daily. Cavaletti Poles 10 repetitions twice daily, High Five 10 repetitions twice daily, Down to Sit 10 repetitions twice daily.

Days 29–56

Focus for management. Continued strengthening.

Pain. Adjust medication as necessary.

Exercise. Twice daily 30 minutes. Off lead for 5 minutes. Introduce mild to moderate hill walking. No games or playing with other dogs.

Modalities. Laser weekly. PEMFT weekly. Hydrotherapy weekly increasing the time in UWTM to a maximum of 20 minutes or therapeutic exercises in the pool building up to a total of 10 minutes swimming.

Therapeutic exercise. Stretches five times twice daily. Cavaletti Poles 15 repetitions twice daily, High Five 15 repetitions three times twice daily. Down to Sit 15 repetitions twice daily. Downhill Walking (Fig. 8.90) 5 minutes twice daily. Play Bow (Fig. 8.36) 15 repetitions twice daily.

Days 57–90

Focus for management. Return to normal activity.

Exercise. Up to 60 minutes walk per day, 15 minutes off lead. Can do moderate to steep hill walking. Gentle ball games (rolling, but not throwing), 5 minutes playing with other dogs.

Modalities. Continue hydrotherapy. Introduce resistance by jets or theraband.

Therapeutic exercise. Continue exercises as mentioned above.

Biceps tendinopathy

In the past, this condition has been overdiagnosed based on a positive biceps stress test. Remember a positive biceps test will also occur with a supraspinatus tendinopathy and a fragmented coronoid process. More often pathology in the biceps tendon is seen as part of other shoulder problems such as medial shoulder instability and supraspinatus tendinopathy.

This condition is seen a lot in agility and fly ball dogs, and also in overweight medium large breeds, for example, Labrador Retrievers.

Signalment. The condition has an insidious onset front-leg lameness varying in severity. There is usually muscle atrophy of supraspinatus. There is pain on palpation of the biceps tendon with shoulder in flexion and elbow in extension. In chronic cases, there may be adaptive shortening of the biceps muscle limiting elbow extension. In severe cases, the biceps tendon will detach completely from the supraglenoid tubercle.

Diagnosis. X-ray with contrast, diagnostic ultrasound, MRI and arthroscopy.

Treatment. Modalities, therapeutic exercise and surgery. Surgery may be indicated for non-responsive dogs or where there has been detachment of the tendon. The installation of platelet-rich plasma and/or stem cells may also be beneficial.

Environmental consideration. The type of flooring should be investigated and any slippery surfaces covered with rugs and runners. Also some sort of ramp or steps should be advised for getting in and out of any vehicle.

Body condition score and diet. A weight-loss program should be instigated for overweight dogs. The addition of EPA to the diet may also be of benefit.

Daily treatment protocols are similar for supraspinatus tendinopathy (see above).

Infraspinatus contracture

This condition is rare and occurs mostly in larger working dogs. Contracture of the infraspinatus muscle causes acute shoulder lameness with outward rotation of the front leg. In the limited number of cases, we have seen, response to shockwave, laser, ultrasound and stretching, and therapeutic exercises has been disappointing. Surgical sectioning of the tendon has been corrective.

Medial shoulder instability

This condition is common in agility and fly ball dogs due to repetitive strain to the shoulder joint. It can also occur in pet animals as a result of slips on laminate or similar flooring.

Signalment. In the pet dog (traumatic case), there is an acute front-leg lameness following a fall. In the canine athlete, the complaint is often refusing tight turns, intermittent lameness becoming more frequent with a poor response to NSAIDS and rest. The whole shoulder area often shows muscle atrophy that can be measured. There is an increased shoulder abduction angle. This should be compared to the contra-lateral leg and careful attention paid to the end feels on each side (Chapter 4). Supraspinatus and biceps tendinopathies are often present.

Diagnosis. Arthroscopy is the method of choice for the confirmation of diagnosis (Figure 11.3). It also allows for the injury to be graded mild, moderate and severe. Mild and moderate cases are usually treated conservatively. Severe cases or poor responders may require surgical stabilisation of the shoulder joint.

Treatment. Mild and moderate cases are normally treated with a combination of a shoulder brace, modalities and therapeutic exercise. The installation of platelet-rich plasma and/or stem cells into the shoulder joint may also be beneficial. For severe cases see at the end of mild and moderate cases protocol.

Mild/Moderate cases

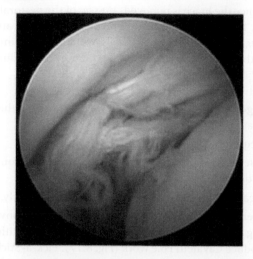

Figure 11.3   Arthroscopy of a shoulder joint showing damage to the medial gleno-humeral ligament.

Days 1–14

Focus for management. Supporting the shoulder joint and preventing further injury. Restarting the inflammatory process. Again as with the shoulder tendinopathies, often the inflammatory response has stopped before healing is complete.

A shoulder brace (DogLeggs) is fitted (Chapter 9). It is important that the brace fits properly and comfortably. A variety of sizes are available. The use of the brace treads a fine line between protecting the joint from further damage through excessive lateral or medial movement whilst still allowing movement and muscle activity in a cranial and caudal direction.

Exercise. Restrict to 15 minutes walk twice daily on the lead in the shoulder brace on level flat round. No games or playing with other dogs.

Pain management. Once again other forms of pain medication should be considered other than NSAIDS.

Environment. Ensure no slippery surfaces and that the patient is lifted in and out of vehicles.

Weight. Management as required.

Modalities. *Shockwave* is the treatment of choice if available. A total of 600–2000 shocks applied around the shoulder. Repeat on day 14. If shockwave is not available, then *laser* around the joint at 12 j/cm^2 at target depth. Repeat every second day. *PEMFT* twice weekly on settings to encourage vascularisation (see manufacturers' instructions).

Therapeutic exercise. These are done with the shoulder brace removed. Passive ROM of the shoulder and elbow, flexion and extension 10 repetitions twice daily. Scapula Mobilisations (Fig. 8.6) for 1 minute twice daily. These are important to prevent fibrosis and the formation of scar tissue that could affect the movement of the scapula once the brace is removed. *Massage* of the pectoral girdle for 5 minutes twice daily. Type of massage will depend on trigger points and tone. Shoulder *joint compressions*, five repetitions twice daily will improve joint health, but care must be taken that there is no medial or lateral movement during compression (Chapter 6).

Days 15–28

Focus for management. Increase in active ROM and strengthening of the supporting musculature.

Pain relief. As required, but still avoiding NSAIDS.

Exercise. Increase lead walks to 20–30 minutes on even ground still with the shoulder brace on. Mild gradients can be introduced.

Modalities. Repeat shockwave on day 28 if using. Laser weekly. PEMFT weekly.

Therapeutic exercise. Continue exercises as mentioned above, but introduce Down to Sit (Fig. 8.33–34) and High Five (Fig. 8.35) 10 repetitions of each twice daily. Also introduce Cavaletti Pole work (Fig. 8.77). Pick-a-Sticks (Fig. 8.78) and Clock Face (Fig. 8.32) all 10 repetitions twice daily. Also introduce Cream Cheese to the Axilla (Fig. 8.37) Three repetitions twice daily. Remove the shoulder brace for this and repeat 10 passes twice daily for each exercise. Also introduce Wobble Cushion (Fig. 8.82) and Rocker Board (Fig. 8.83) 30 seconds twice daily on each.

Days 29–60

Focus for management. Strengthening.

Exercise. Twice daily 30–45 minutes walk on lead but out of shoulder brace. Introduce moderate hills. Dog can be off lead for 5 minutes on each walk, but no games or playing with other dogs.

Modalities. Continue laser and PEMFT weekly.

Therapeutic exercise. Continue with exercises from above but increase repetitions by 50%. Introduce Side Stepping 3 m (10 ft) in both directions three repetitions twice (Fig. 8.95) Figures of Eight (Fig. 8.81) five repetitions twice daily.

Days 61–90

Focus for management. Increased strengthening and return to normal activities.

Exercise. Twice daily 60 minutes walk, out of the shoulder brace, off lead for 20 minutes. Low-impact games, for example, rolling a ball. Limited interaction with other dogs provided not too rough.

Modalities. Hydrotherapy weekly as mentioned above.

Therapeutic exercise. As mentioned above, but increase repetitions by another 50%.

Severe cases or non-responders that go to surgery are often placed in a Velpeau sling for the first 14 days post operation.

Days 1–14

Focus for management. Wound management with icing for 10 minutes twice daily.

Pain relief. Opiates or other pain medication, but try to avoid NSAIDS.

Exercise. Strict rest with toilet breaks only.

Modalities. Laser 12 j/cm² at target tissue every other day. PEMFT set on pain relief (see manufacturers' settings) daily.

Therapeutic exercise. Passive ROM, flexion and extension of elbow, carpus and digits, six repetitions twice daily (Figs. 8.7–9, 8.15–6).

After the first 2 weeks, the severe cases will follow a similar protocol as for the mild and moderate cases, starting at day 1. Recovery will be slower and regular reassessments are vital.

As with all the suggested protocols, there will be great variation from patient to patient and the protocols are meant only as a guide. The clinician must assess each case regularly and make adjustments to the protocol accordingly.

Elbow

Elbows can be difficult joints to rehabilitate. Common problems are contracture of the flexor tendons, atrophy of triceps muscles and a reduction in ROM. Early physiotherapy interventions are essential to prevent the above happening, but the treatment plan must also take into account any surgical procedure that has been performed.

Fragmented coronoid process

This a common condition in the elbow of certain breeds, for example, Bernese Mountain Dog, Labrador Retriever and Rottweiler. A fragment of the medial ulna coronoid process breaks off or fissures.

Signalment. An insidious onset front-leg lameness in dogs less than 12 months of age. Some FCPs do not present until much later in life when the effects of the osteoarthritis caused by the FCP become apparent. Lameness can be mild to severe and can be bilateral. These dogs will have a positive biceps stress test. There can be a significant muscle atrophy.

Diagnosis. X-ray, CT and arthroscopy (Figure 11.4).

Treatment. Conservative management, arthroscopic removal of fragments and biceps ulna release procedure (BURP). Other more involved surgical techniques have also been described for extensive cartilage damage, for example, proximal abducting ulna osteotomy (PAUL).

Surgical cases (Arthroscopic removal of fragment, BURP).

Conservative management would start at day 15.

Days 1–5

Focus for management. Wound care, post-operative swelling. Pain control. Avoiding flexor tendon contracture.

Pain relief. NSAIDS and opiates as required.

Environment. Check type of flooring and advise rugs and runners as required.

Diet. Advise weight loss if overweight. Consider the addition of EPA to ration.

Exercise. Restricted to short toilet breaks on the lead. No stairs. No games or playing with other dogs.

Modalities. Icing to elbow for 10 minutes twice daily. Every other day, laser 5 j/cm² at target tissue applied around the joint line but paying particular

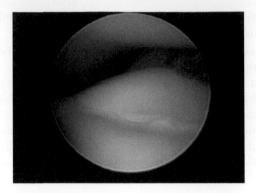

Figure 11.4 Arthroscopy of an elbow showing flap of cartilage from the coronoid process of ulna.

attention to the medial compartment. PEMFT 20 minutes daily set for pain relief (see manufacturers' guidelines).

Therapeutic exercise. Perform passive ROM of the elbow, starting with flexion, (Fig. 8.7) five repetitions twice daily and progressing to extension as well, (Fig. 8.8) when dog comfortable enough. Passive flexion and extension of shoulder, carpus and digits. Five repetitions twice daily (Figs. 8.2–3, 8.9–10, 8.15–16).

Days 6–14

Focus for management. Maintaining/increasing ROM of elbow. Prevention of flexor tendon contracture.

Pain relief. NSAIDS.

Exercise. Walk for 5 minutes on lead on level flat ground. No games or playing with other dogs. No stairs.

Modalities. Laser twice weekly. PEMFT twice weekly set to encourage blood supply (see manufacturers' guidelines).

Therapeutic exercise. Passive flexion and extension of elbow, 10 repetitions twice daily. Passive flexion and extension of shoulder, carpus and digits as mentioned above. Stretch of triceps by flexing elbow and extending shoulder. Repeat five times twice daily (Fig. 8.49).

Days 15–30

Focus for management. Active range of motion. Early strengthening.

Pain relief. Continue NSAIDS.

Exercise. Twice daily 10 minutes on the lead. Can introduce gentle gradients. No games or playing with other dogs. No stairs.

Modalities. Continue laser and PEMFT at weekly intervals. Introduce hydrotherapy twice weekly. Just cover the feet with water if using UWTM. Go at a slow speed to encourage active ROM with full flexion and extension of all the front-leg joints. Gradually increase session interval from 3 to 20 minutes. If in pool, carry out flexion and extension, and weight shifting exercise on platforms.

Again gradually build up length of time in the water and introduce short spells of assisted swimming.

Therapeutic exercises. Cavaletti Pole work (Fig. 8.77). Twice daily 10 repetitions. High Five (Fig. 8.35) 5 repetitions twice daily. Down to a Sit (Fig. 8.33–34), five repetitions twice daily. Rebounding (Fig. 8.76) for 2 minutes twice daily. Figures of Eight (Fig. 8.81), five repetitions twice daily.

Days 30–60

Focus for management. Strengthening.

Pain relief. NSAIDS as required.

Exercise. Walk 20 minutes twice daily and 5 minutes off lead. Moderate hill work. Low-impact games, such as rolling a ball. No playing with other dogs.

Modalities. Hydrotherapy weekly. Increase depth of water to cover the elbow if using UWTM. Increase speed. If in the pool, introduce free swimming and gradually increase to 10 minutes.

Therapeutic exercise. Continue exercises as for days 15–30, but increase repetitions by 100%, except for the Cavaletti poles. Raise the Cavaletti poles using blocks or drinks cans (Fig. 8.102). Do 15 passes twice daily.

Days 61–90

Focus for management. Return to normal activities.

Pain relief. NSAIDS as required.

Exercise. Walk 45 minutes twice daily. Off lead for 20 minutes. Gentle games and playing with other dogs.

Modalities. Hydrotherapy weekly as mentioned above.

Therapeutic exercise. As for days 30–60, but increase repetitions by 50%.

Other elbow conditions such as ununited anconeal process, osteochondrosis, incomplete ossification of humeral condyles (IOHC), condylar fractures, will mostly be treated surgically. Attention must be paid to the type and stability of the repair when drawing up a treatment plan. Position of implants must also be considered when using modalities such as laser. Also bear in mind that flexor tendon contracture, triceps atrophy and reduced elbow ROM are the common sequels to elbow surgery.

Carpus

Hyperextension injury. This is relatively a common condition and can be seen as a result of a single dramatic traumatic event or from repetitive strains.

Signalment. Hyperextension of the carpus, usually greater than 30° past the normal range. The dog may even walk on the palmer surface of the carpus.

Diagnosis. X-ray – may need stressed views. The condition is graded 1–3 depending upon severity.

Treatment. Grade 1 and 2 may respond to the use of a carpal support (Chapter 9) but may also benefit from the use of platelet-rich plasma and/or stem cells. Grade 3 injuries and poor responders are usually treated by pancarpal arthrodesis.

Protocol for pancarpal arthrodesis

Days 1–5 (Figure 11.5)

Focus for management. Wound care, post-operative swelling and pain control.

Pain relief. NSAIDS and opiates as required.

Environment. Check type of flooring and advise rugs and runners as required.

Diet. Advise weight loss if overweight. Consider the addition of EPA to ration.

Exercise. Restricted to short toilet breaks on the lead. No stairs. No games or playing with other dogs.

Modalities. These dogs may have a splint on. The modalities would be carried out at a splint change before the new splint or dressing is applied. Icing to carpus for 10 minutes twice daily. Every other day laser 5 j/cm² at target tissue. Avoid the plate, as it will absorb the laser beam. PEMFT 20 minutes daily set for pain relief (see manufacturers' guidelines).

Therapeutic exercise. Perform passive ROM of the shoulder, elbow and digits. Five repetitions twice daily (Figs. 8.2–3, 8.7–8, 8.15–16).

Days 6–14

Focus for management. Protection of the arthrodesis surgery. Prevention of shortening of biceps and triceps.

Pain relief. NSAIDS.

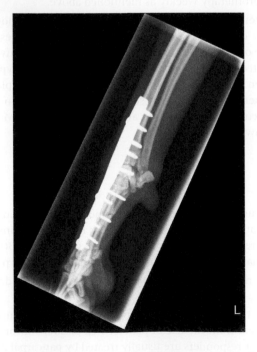

Figure 11.5   Post-operative X-ray of a pancarpal arthrodesis.

Exercise. Walk 5 minutes on lead on level flat ground. No games or playing with other dogs. No stairs.

Modalities. Laser twice weekly. PEMFT twice weekly set to encourage blood supply (see manufacturers' guidelines).

Therapeutic exercise. Passive flexion and extension of shoulder, elbow and digits. Ten repetitions twice daily. Stretch of triceps by flexing elbow and extending shoulder. Stretch of biceps by flexing shoulder and extension of the elbow (Fig. 8.49). Repeat three times twice daily.

Days 15–45

Focus for management. Protection of arthrodesis surgery. Prevention of muscle atrophy.

Pain relief. Continue NSAIDS.

Exercise. Gradually build up to 15 minutes walk twice daily on the lead. Gentle gradients can be introduced. No games or playing with other dogs. No stairs.

Modalities. Continue laser and PEMFT at weekly intervals.

Therapeutic exercises. Continue passive ROM exercises and stretches as for days 6–14. Rebounding (Fig. 8.76) for 2 minutes twice daily. Figures of Eight (Fig. 8.81), five repetitions twice daily.

Days 46–90

Focus for management. Active ROM. Strengthening.

Pain relief. NSAIDS as required.

Exercise. Walk 20 minutes twice daily on lead. Moderate hill work. No games or playing with other dogs.

Modalities. Introduce hydrotherapy weekly. Initially just cover the feet with water to encourage active flexion and extension of the joints. Gradually increase depth of water to cover the elbow if using UWTM. Increase speed. If in the pool, do therapeutic exercises on platforms and start free swimming.

Therapeutic exercise. Continue Rebounding and Figures of Eight. Introduce Cavaletti Poles (Fig. 8.77). 10 passes twice daily. Also introduce High Five (Fig. 8.35) and Down to Sit (fig. 8.33–4) exercises, 10 repetitions twice daily.

Days 90–120

Focus for management. Return to normal activities.

Pain relief. NSAIDS as required.

Exercise. Walk 45 minutes twice daily. Off lead for 10 minutes. Gentle games and playing with other dogs.

Modalities. Hydrotherapy weekly as mentioned above.

Therapeutic exercise. As for days 46–90, but increase repetitions by 50%.

Hip

Hip dysplasia

This is the most commonly diagnosed orthopaedic problem in the growing dog. The disease is multifactorial with breed, lifestyle and diet all playing a part.

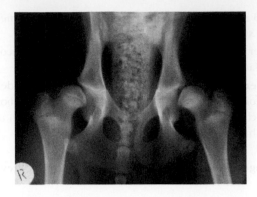

Figure 11.6   Radiograph of a young dog with hip dysplasia.

Signalment. Young dog that wants to sit down a lot. The dog may sit with its back legs to one side. At a walk, there is usually a swaggering gait. The dog uses the iliopsoas and paraspinal muscles to advance the pelvic leg rather than flex and extend the hip joint. Hip extension is resented. There is likely to be muscle wasting of the gluteal, quadriceps and hamstring muscles.

Diagnosis. X-ray (Figure 11.6).

Treatment. Many surgical procedures have been described for the treatment of HD in the young dog. These include triple- and double-pelvic osteotomies and juvenile pelvic symphysiodesis. One of the authors (DP) prefers to manage these dogs conservatively until they are 10–12 months of age. If they are still lame at this stage, then a total hip replacement is recommended. The rationale behind this protocol is that many of these dogs will improve without the need for surgery. The reversal of the muscle atrophy is important in this respect and if the patient is subsequently referred for THR, the increased muscle mass will be of benefit post operatively. Also, THRs have a good success rate in the hands of the correct surgeon. The prosthetic hips now last well beyond the lifespan of a dog and so the problem of having to replace a worn out hip prosthesis does not usually occur.

Conservative management

Days 1–14

Focus for management. Pain relief. Joint health.

Pain relief. NSAIDS +/− adjunct as required.

Environment. Check what type of flooring and advise rugs and runners as required. Advise the use of ramps for getting in and out of vehicles. Advise deep soft bedding. These dogs spend a lot of time lying down and often chose hard surfaces. Try to avoid these as calluses or decubit ulcers may arise.

Diet. These dogs are doing much less active and may put on weight if the amount of food is not adjusted.

Exercise. On lead for 5–10 minutes twice daily on flat level ground. No stairs. No games or playing with other dogs.

Modalities. Laser 5 j/cm^2 at target tissue twice weekly (Chapter 5). Laser hip joint and iliopsoas muscles. PEMFT set for pain relief (see manufacturers' guidelines) for 20 minutes twice daily (Chapter 5). EMS to gluteal muscles, quads and hamstrings for 10 minutes every other day (Chapter 5). Hydrotherapy twice weekly (Chapter 5). If using UWTM, fill to mid femur and slowly walk for 3 minutes gradually building up to 10 minutes. If using pool stand on platforms, perform therapeutic exercises. Start assisted swimming gradually building up to 5 minutes.

Therapeutic exercise. Joint compressions five repetitions twice daily (Chapter 6). Passive flexion and extension of hip, stifle, hock and digits repeated three times twice daily (Figs. 8.15–18, 8.21–24). Iliopsoas Stretch repeated three times twice daily (Fig. 8.52). Tug of War High Up (Fig. 8.98). Do for 2 minutes twice daily. This is a good exercise as the young dog gets to play without much movement of the hip joint. Rebounding for 2 minutes twice daily (Fig. 8.76). Also fine balance movements, such as Standing on Air Mattress (Fig. 8.66) or Wobble Cushion (Fig. 8.82) for 1 minute, repeated twice daily.

Days 15–45

Focus for management. Pain relief. Active ROM. Early strengthening.

Pain relief. NSAIDS.

Exercise. Twice daily 10–15 minutes on lead. Can introduce gentle gradients. No stairs. No games or playing with other dogs.

Modalities. Continue laser and PEMFT weekly. Continue hydrotherapy weekly. If using UWTM, gradually increase session length to 20 minutes. Vary water height to encourage active flexion and extension of back leg joints. This also reduces the buoyancy. If in pool, introduce free swimming. Continue with therapeutic exercises.

Therapeutic exercise. Continue therapeutic exercises as per days 1–14, but increase repetitions by 50%. Add the following exercises: Cream Cheese to the Groin (Fig. 8.40) three repetitions twice daily, Biscuits from Hips (Fig. 8.29) and Sit to Stand (Fig. 39–40) both 10 repetitions twice daily. Backwards Walking (Fig. 8.100) 10 ft repeated three times twice daily.

Days 46–90

Focus for management. Pain relief. Strengthening.

Pain relief. Continue NSAIDS as required.

Exercise. Lead walk 30–45 minutes. Off lead for 5 minutes. Introduce moderate gradients. Introduce stairs gradually. No games or playing with other dogs.

Modalities. Continue as per days 15–45.

Therapeutic exercise. Iliopsoas stretch repeated three times twice daily. Tug of War High Up for 5 minutes twice daily. Biscuits from the Hips, Sit to Stand, both 15 repetitions three times daily. Backwards Walking, 20 ft repeated five times thrice daily. Three-leg standing for 1 minute on each leg repeated three times twice daily (Fig. 8.62). Standing with Front Legs on Swiss Ball (Fig. 8.96) for 2 minutes repeated three times twice daily.

Days 91–120

Focus for management. Return to normal activity.

Pain relief. NSAIDS as required.

Exercise. Lead walk 45–60 minutes twice daily. Allow off lead for 10 minutes of each walk. Introduce varied terrain and steeper hills. Start low-impact games, for example, ball rolling. Allow 5 minutes play with other dogs twice daily.

Modalities. Fortnightly hydrotherapy.

Therapeutic exercise. As per days 45–90, but increase repetitions by 50%.

Femoral head osteotomy (FHO)

This is a salvage procedure where the femoral head is removed, and hence there is no articulation between the pelvis and the femur. Early post-operative rehabilitation is aimed at weight bearing as soon as possible (Figure 11.7).

Days 1–5

Focus for management. Pain relief and wound management.

Pain relief. NSAIDS +/– Opiates.

Environment. Check for suitable flooring and bedding.

Diet. Weight loss if required.

Exercise. Twice daily 5 minutes on lead on level even ground. No games or playing with other dogs and no stairs.

Modalities. Icing to wound 10 minutes twice daily. Laser 5 j/cm^2 at osteotomy site every other day. PEMFT set for pain relief (see manufacturers' instructions), 20 minutes every other day.

Therapeutic exercise. Passive range of motion, flexion and extension of stifle, hock and digits, (Figs. 8.21–24, 8.15–16) three repetitions twice daily.

Days 6–14

Focus for management. Pain relief, early weight bearing.

Pain relief. NSAIDS.

Exercise. Build up to 10 minutes on lead on level even ground. No games or playing with other dogs, and no stairs.

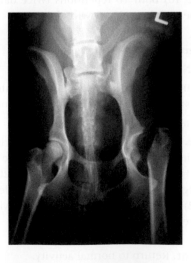

Figure 11.7   Post-operative X-ray of a femoral head osteotomy.

Modalities. Laser and PEMF as for days 1–5. EMS 10 minutes twice weekly to gluteals.

Therapeutic exercise. Passive ROM as for days 1–5. Introduce Cream Cheese to the Groin (Fig. 8.40) three repetitions twice daily. Parastanding 1 Book (Fig. 8.58) 30 seconds three times twice daily both with affected and unaffected leg on the book sequentially.

Days 15–30

Focus for management. Weight bearing. Active ROM.

Pain relief. NSAIDS as required.

Exercise. Build up to 20 minutes on lead. Introduce mild hill work. No games or playing with other dogs. Can start to attempt stairs.

Modalities. Laser and PEMFT weekly. EMS to gluteals twice weekly. Introduce hydrotherapy. In this case, the UWTM is far better than the pool as water depth and speed can be carefully controlled. Start with water just below the hip for maximum buoyancy. Gradually build up to 10 minutes twice weekly.

Therapeutic exercise. Continue book parastanding as per days 6–14 but double the time and repetitions. Introduce Rebounding (Fig. 8.76) 30 seconds twice daily, 3 Leg Standing (Fig. 8.61) 30 seconds twice daily, Cavaletti Poles (Fig. 8.77) five repetitions twice daily, and Standing on Air Mattress (Fig. 8.66) 1 minute twice daily.

Days 30–60

Focus for management. Strengthening.

Pain relief. NSAIDS as required.

Exercise. Walk 30 minutes twice daily. Allow off lead for 5 minutes each walk. Introduce moderate hills. No games or playing with other dogs.

Modalities. Hydrotherapy (UWTM) weekly. Gradually increase time to 20 minutes per session and decrease water level to below stifle.

Therapeutic exercise. Continue exercises as per days 15–30 but double repetitions/time. Introduce Sit to Stand (Fig. 8.38–9) 10 repetitions twice daily, Backwards Walking (Fig. 8.100) 10 repetitions twice daily.

Days 61–120

Focus for management. Further strengthening. Return to normal activity.

Exercise. Build up to 45–60 minutes walk on lead twice daily. Allow off lead for 15 each walk. Introduce low-impact games, such as ball rolling and playing with other dogs.

Modalities. Continue hydrotherapy (UWTM) as per days 30–60 weekly.

Therapeutic exercise. Sit to Stand and Backwards Walking, 15 repetitions three times daily.

Total hip replacement (THR)

With most THRs, the dog improves dramatically as the pain is removed. In these cases, care needs to be taken to have controlled exercise and not to jeopardise the surgery. This should continue for the first 4–6 weeks until there is radiographic evidence of new bone growth into the implant (Figure 11.8).

Days 1–14

Focus for management. Pain relief and wound management.

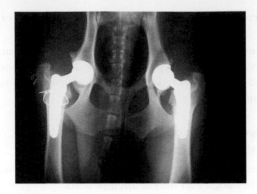

Figure 11.8 Post-operative X-ray of a total hip replacement.

Pain relief. NSAIDS +/− opiates.

Environment. Check suitability of flooring and bedding.

Diet. Weight loss as required.

Exercise. Toilet breaks on lead only twice daily. Restricted activity.

Modalities. Icing to wound 10 minutes twice daily.

Therapeutic exercise. Passive ROM, extension and flexion of stifle, hock and digits. (Figs. 8.21–24, 8.15–16) Three repetitions twice daily.

Days 15–45

Focus for management. Protection of surgery.

Pain relief. NSAIDS as required.

Exercise. Gradually build up to 10 minutes on the lead twice daily on flat even ground. No games, no stairs and no playing with other dogs.

Therapeutic exercise. Continue passive ROM as per days 1–14.

Days 46–90

Focus for management. Strengthening.

Exercise. Gradually build up to 20 minutes lead walk twice daily. Introduce mild gradients. No games or playing with other dogs and no stairs.

Modalities. Introduce hydrotherapy. Again the UWTM gives more control with depth of water and speed. Start with the water just above feet to encourage active ROM. Build sessions gradually to 15 minutes. Gradually increase depth of water to above the stifle. Alternatively introduce assisted swimming for short periods. Gradually build to 2–5minutes unassisted swimming.

Therapeutic exercise. Cavaletti Poles (Fig. 8.77) 10 repetitions twice daily, Sit to Stand (Fig. 8.38–9) and Backwards walking (Fig. 8.100) both 10 repetitions twice daily.

Days 91–120

Focus for management. Further strengthening and return to normal activity.

Exercise. Gradually build walks to 45 minutes twice daily. Allow off lead for 5 minutes during each walk. Introduce moderate hills.

Modalities. Continue hydrotherapy gradually increasing session length to 20 minutes.

Therapeutic exercise. As per days 46–90 but increase repetitions to 15 three times daily.

Gracilis myopathy

This condition mainly occurs in working dogs, particularly German Shepherds although we do see a significant number in agility dogs. Aetiology is unknown but repetitive strain, ischaemia and autoimmune causes have all been suggested. The condition may also involve the semi-membranosus, semi-tendinosus and adductor muscles. Normal muscle fibres are replaced by fibrotic scar tissue. This produces a typical diagnostic gait. In early cases, swelling of the muscle belly may be palpated on the caudo-medial thigh. In chronic cases, a taut band of scar tissue replaces this swelling.

Treatment. Surgical options have proved mostly unsuccessful.

Conservative rehabilitation

Acute case

Days 1–21

Focus for management. Pain relief. Reduction in swelling. Prevention of scar tissue formation.

Pain relief. NSAIDS.

Environment. Check flooring and vehicle entry and exit.

Exercise. Walk 5 minute on lead on level even ground twice daily. No games or playing with other dogs, and no stairs.

Modalities. Icing 10 minutes twice daily. Ultrasound. 3.3 MHz (or 1 MHz if adductor involved) 20% pulsed, 2.0 W/cm^2 intensity for 5 minutes over the muscle belly and tendon, repeated every other day.

Therapeutic exercise. Gracilis Stretch (Fig. 8.54) three repetitions twice daily. Backwards Walking (Fig. 8.100) for 3 m (10 ft) repeated three times twice daily. Massage (Chapter 6) 5 minutes twice daily.

Days 22–45

Focus for management. Prevention of scar tissue formation.

Pain relief. NSAIDS as required.

Exercise. 15 minutes twice daily on lead. Introduce mild inclines and declines and traversing gentle slope faces. No games or playing with other dogs.

Modalities. Continue pulsed ultrasound weekly. Introduce hydrotherapy with assisted swimming for 5 minutes or UWTM with water above the stifle for 5 minutes.

Therapeutic exercise. Continue as per days 1–21 but increase repetitions to three times daily. Introduce Side Stepping (Fig. 8.95) 3 m (10 ft) repeated three times twice daily.

Chronic case

Days 1–14

Focus for management. Increase in elasticity of scar tissue.

Pain relief. Acetaminophen (paracetamol), tramadol.

Exercise. Twice daily 20 minutes on the lead. Moderate hill work including traversing.

Modalities. Day 1. Shockwave 800–2000 shocks over the muscle belly and full length of the tendon.

Manual therapies. Cross-frictional massage 3 minutes twice daily (Chapter 6).

Therapeutic exercise. Gracilis Stretch (Fig. 8.54) three repetitions twice daily. Backwards Walking (Fig. 8.100) for 3 m (10 ft) repeated three times twice daily. Side Stepping (Fig. 8.95) 3 m (10 ft) repeated three times twice daily.

Days 15–22

Focus for management. As per days 1–14.

Pain relief. As per days 1–14.

Exercise. Lead walk 30 minutes twice daily. Introduce steeper hills.

Modalities. Repeat shockwave on days 15 and 22. Introduce hydrotherapy. This is best done in the UWTM. Water above stifle building to 15 minutes weekly.

Manual therapies. Cross-frictional massage 5 minutes three times daily.

Therapeutic exercise. As per days 1–14, but increase repetitions to three times daily.

Days 23–90

Focus for management. As per day 1.

Modalities. Continue hydrotherapy. Introduce PEMFT 20 minutes twice weekly set for increase in vascularity (see manufactures' instructions). Introduce continuous ultrasound 3.3 MHz (1 MHz if adductor involved) intensity 1.5 W/cm² for 5 minutes repeated twice weekly.

Manual therapies. As per days 15–22.

Therapeutic exercise. As per days 15–22.

Stifle
Cranial cruciate ligament rupture

Signalment. This is one of the most common orthopaedic conditions encountered in practice. Most ruptures are a slow degeneration of the ligament but often present as sudden-onset lameness when full rupture occurs. Presenting signs are toe touching or non-weight bearing on the affected leg. Joint effusion and a medial buttress on proximal tibia are usually present. Muscle wasting of the quadriceps and hamstrings when compared to the contra-lateral side is also a common feature. A high percentage of cases are or go on to be bilateral. Many will have meniscal damage.

Diagnosis. The demonstration of a cranial drawer (the patient may need to be sedated or anaesthetised for this) X-ray, arthroscopy and MRI.

Treatment. Most cases are better managed surgically. Surgical management allows investigation and addressing of any meniscal injury as well as debridement of the ruptured ligament. Over the years, many surgical techniques have been described. Currently three techniques are currently popular: a lateral suture, a tibial plateau levelling osteotomy (TPLO) and a tibial tuberosity advancement (TTA). The latter two involve osteotomies of the tibia and placement of plates and screws. The position of the plate and screws as well as the time taken for the osteotomy sites to heal are important considerations of any rehabilitation program. Whilst surgery would be the first choice for management, there may be situations where other health or financial issues may result in a request for conservative management.

Conservative management. In some dogs, this can take a long time, longer than surgical cases. If a meniscal injury is present, these dogs may never be sound.

Days 1–14

Focus for management. Pain relief. Joint health. Increasing weight bearing.

Pain relief. NSAIDS

Environment. Check flooring and use rugs and runners as required.

Diet. Weight loss as required. Ensure inclusion of EPA to the diet.

Exercise. 5 minutes on lead on even level ground. No games or playing with other dogs or stairs.

Modalities. Laser 8 j/cm^2 at the target area. Laser around the joint line. Repeat twice weekly. PEMFT 20 minutes twice weekly set for pain relief (see manufacturers' instructions.) Hydrotherapy twice weekly. If using UWTM, start with 4-minute sessions with water above the stifle. Gradually build the session intervals to 10 minutes. If using pool, perform therapeutic exercises on platforms and start assisted swimming. Gradually build to 10 minutes free swimming.

Manual therapies. Joint compressions five repetitions twice daily. Grade 1 and 2 joint mobilisations three repetitions twice daily.

Therapeutic exercise. PROM, flexion and extension of hip, hock and digits (Figs. 88.17–18, 8.23–24, 8.15–16) three repetitions twice daily. Parastanding 1 Book (Fig. 8.58) 30 seconds three times daily with affected and unaffected leg on the book.

Days 15–30

Focus for management. Increase weight bearing, core stability and early strengthening.

Pain relief. NSAIDS.

Exercise. 10 minutes on lead twice daily. No games or playing with other dogs or stairs.

Modalities. Laser and PEMFT weekly, settings as above. Continue with weekly hydrotherapy gradually increasing session length to 20 minutes.

Manual therapies. Continue joint compressions as above. Move onto Grade 3 joint mobilisations, three repetitions twice daily (Chapter 6).

Therapeutic exercise. Biscuits from Hips (Fig. 8.29) 10 repetitions twice daily to both sides. Sit to Stand (Fig. 8.38–9) 10 repetitions twice daily. Backwards Walking (Fig. 8.100) 3 m (10 ft) three repetitions twice daily. Rebounding (fig. 8.76) 2 minutes twice daily. 3 Leg Standing Back Leg (Fig. 8.62) 30 seconds twice daily.

Days 31–120

Focus for management. Strengthening.

Pain relief. NSAIDS.

Exercise. 20–30 minutes lead exercise twice daily. Allow off lead for 5 minutes twice daily. Introduce mild and moderate gradients. Introduce stairs. No games or playing with other dogs.

Modalities. Laser and hydrotherapy weekly as above.

Manual therapies. Grade 3 or 4 joint mobilisations as required, three repetitions weekly.

Therapeutic exercise. As per days 15–30, but increase repetition by 50%.

Days 121–180

Focus for management. Strengthening and return to normal activity.

Pain relief. NSAIDS as required.

Exercise. 30–45 minutes lead walk. Off lead for 15 minutes. Introduce steep hills. Traverse as well as going up and down. Gentle ball games. Playing for 5 minutes with other dogs.

Modalities. As per days 31–120.

Therapeutic exercise. As per days 31–120, but increase repetitions by 50%.

Surgical management
Lateral suture

Post operative rehabilitation. Days 1–14

Focus for management. Pain relief. Post-operative swelling. Wound management. PROM.

Pain relief. NSAIDS +/− opiates.

Environment. Check flooring and access points. Introduce rugs, runners and ramps as required.

Diet. Weight loss as required. Include EPA in diet.

Exercise. 5 minutes on lead on even level ground. No games or playing with other dogs, and no stairs.

Modalities. Icing 10 minutes twice daily for first 5 days. Laser 8 j/cm^2 at the target area. Laser around the joint line. Repeat twice weekly. PEMFT 20 minutes twice weekly set for pain relief (see manufacturers' instructions). EMS to quads and hamstrings set to synchronised 10 minutes every other day (Chapter 5).

Manual therapies. Joint compressions five repetitions twice daily. Grade 1 and 2 joint mobilisations three repetitions twice daily. three repetitions twice daily (Chapter 6).

Therapeutic exercise. PROM, flexion and extension of hip, hock and digits (Figs. 8.8.16–7, 8.23–4, 8.15–6) three repetitions twice daily.

Days 15–30

Focus for management. Early weight bearing, core stability and reversal of muscle loss.

Pain relief. NSAIDS

Exercise. 10 minutes on lead on level even ground. No games or playing with other dogs, and no stairs.

Modalities. Laser and PEMFT weekly using setting as for days 1–14. Introduce hydrotherapy. Hydrotherapy twice weekly. If using UWTM, start with 4-minute sessions with water above the stifle. Gradually build the session length to 10 minutes. If using pool, perform therapeutic exercises on platforms and start assisted swimming. Gradually build to 10 minutes free swimming.

Manual therapies. Continue joint compressions above. Move onto Grade 3 joint mobilisations, three repetitions twice daily.

Therapeutic exercise. Biscuits from Hips (Fig. 8.29) 10 repetitions twice daily to both sides. Sit to Stand (Fig. 8.38–9) 10 repetitions twice daily. Backwards Walking (Fig. 8.100) 3 m (10 ft) three repetitions twice daily. Rebounding (Fig. 8.76) 2 minutes twice daily. 3 Leg Standing Back Leg (Fig. 8.62) 30 seconds twice daily.

Days 31–60

Focus for management. Strengthening.

Pain relief. NSAIDS.

Exercise. 20–30 minutes lead exercise twice daily. Introduce mild and moderate gradients. Introduce stairs. No games or playing with other dogs.

Modalities. Laser and PEMFT weekly, settings as above. Continue with weekly hydrotherapy gradually increasing session length to 20 minutes.

Manual therapies. Joint mobilisations as required.

Therapeutic exercise. As per days 15–30, but increase repetitions by 50%.

Days 61–90

Focus for management. Further strengthening and return to normal activity.

Pain relief. NSAIDS as required.

Exercise. 30–45 minutes lead walk. Off lead for 15 minutes. Introduce steep hills. Traverse as well as going up and down. Gentle ball games. 5 minutes playing with other dogs.

Modalities. As per days 31–60.

Therapeutic exercise. As per days 31–60, but increase repetitions by 50%.

Post operation Rehabilitation

TPLO, TTA (Figures 11.9 and 11.10).

Days 1–14 as per lateral suture mentioned above. Laser osteotomy site as well but approach from lateral side to avoid implants.

Days 15–45

Focus for management. Protection of implants. Early weight bearing, core stability and reversal of muscle loss.

Pain relief. NSAIDS.

Exercise. 10 minutes on lead on level even ground. No games or playing with other dogs, and no stairs.

Modalities. Laser and PEMFT weekly using setting as for days 1–14. Continue EMS twice weekly.

Manual therapies. Continue joint compressions above.

Therapeutic exercise. Biscuits from Hips (Fig. 8.29) Parastanding 1 Book (Fig. 8.58) 30 seconds twice daily with affected and unaffected leg on book.

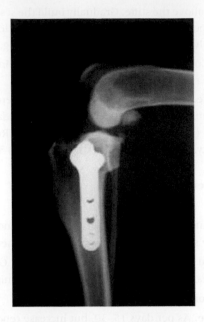

Figure 11.9   Post-operative X-ray of a tibial plateau levelling osteotomy.

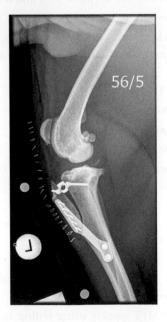

Figure 11.10   Post-operative X-ray of a tibial tuberosity advancement.

Days 46–90

Focus for management. Healing of osteotomy site and strengthening.

Check X-rays taken at this period should demonstrate adequate healing of osteotomy site. If healing is not satisfactory, consider laser at settings 12 j/cm^2 at the target depth every other day for 2 weeks. Alternatively, use shockwave to the osteotomy site 500–1500 shocks. Repeat in 14 days.

If osteotomy wound healing is satisfactory follow below.

Exercise. 20–30 minutes lead exercise twice daily. Introduce mild and moderate gradients. Introduce stairs. No games or playing with other dogs.

Modalities. Laser and PEMFT weekly using setting as for days 1–14. Introduce hydrotherapy. Hydrotherapy twice weekly. If using UWTM, start with 4-minute sessions with water above the stifle. Gradually build the session length to 10 minutes. If using pool, perform therapeutic exercises on platforms and start assisted swimming. Gradually build to 10 minutes free swimming.

Manual therapies. Joint mobilisations. Three repetitions twice daily.

Therapeutic exercise. Biscuits from Hips 10 repetitions twice daily to both sides. Sit to Stand 10 repetitions twice daily. Backwards Walking 3 m (10 ft) three repetitions twice daily. Rebounding 2 minutes twice daily. 3 Leg Standing Back Leg 30 seconds twice daily

Days 91–120

Focus for management. Further strengthening and return to normal activity.

Pain relief. NSAIDS as required.

Exercise. 30–45 minutes lead walk. Off lead for 15 minutes. Introduce steep hills. Traverse as well as going up and down. Gentle ball games. 5 minutes playing with other dogs.

Modalities. As per days 31–60.

Therapeutic exercise. As per days 31–60, but increase repetitions by 50%.

Medial patella luxation

This is a common developmental problem in smaller breeds such as Yorkshire Terriers and Pugs. It also occurs in Labrador Retrievers. The dog may hop occasionally or carry the leg completely depending on severity. There may be angular deformities of the femur and tibia.

Diagnosis. Clinical examination, X-ray and CT scan.

Treatment. Patella luxations are graded 1–4 depending on severity. Grade 1 and non-lame grade 2 luxations respond well to conservative management. While a lot of dogs will 'live' with the condition, the lameness can suddenly deteriorate. This may be due to an increase in the severity of osteoarthritis in the joint or the development of cruciate disease. These require surgery. Various techniques have been described. The most commonly used is a tibial tuberosity transplant, +/– sulcoplasty, +/– capsular overlay.

Conservative management. Grades 1 and 2a.

Days 1–45

Focus for management. Strengthening of quadriceps and lateral thigh muscles (biceps femoris and tensor fascia lata) and reducing outward rotation of hip if present.

Pain relief. None.

Environment. Check flooring and access points. Introduce rugs, runners and ramps as required.

Diet. Weight loss as required. Include EPA in diet.

Exercise. 45–60 minutes lead walk. Introduce moderate and steep inclines. Off lead for 10 minutes each walk. Stairs are allowed but no games or playing with other dogs.

Modalities. Hydrotherapy. Build up to 15-minute sessions in the UWTM with the water above the stifle.

Manual therapies. Flex and extend stifle while holding the patella in the trochlear groove. Repeat 10 times twice daily.

Therapeutic exercise. Theraband tied in such a way as to internally rotate stifle and produce resistance to quadriceps (Fig. 8.104–7) Walk for 5 minutes twice daily gradually building up to 15 minutes twice daily in theraband. Wobble cushion (Fig. 8.82) for 1 minute twice daily gradually increasing to 5 minutes twice daily. Theraband can also be worn for this exercise. The theraband can also be worn in the UWTM Side Stepping (Fig. 8.95) for 3 m (10 ft) repeated three times twice daily. Progress to Sideways walking uphill and gradually increasing the gradient.

Surgical management for grades II, III, 1V (Figure 11.11).

Post operation. Days 1–14

Focus for management. Pain relief. Post-operative swelling. Wound management. PROM.

Pain relief. NSAIDS +/− opiates.

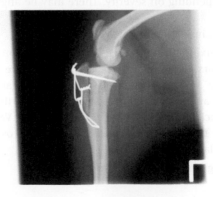

Figure 11.11   Post-operative X-ray of a tibial tuberosity transplant.

Environment. Check flooring and access points. Introduce rugs, runners and ramps as required.

Diet. Weight loss as required. Include EPA in diet.

Exercise. 5 minutes on lead on even level ground. No games or playing with other dogs, and no stairs.

Modalities. Icing 10 minutes twice daily for first 5 days. Laser 8 j/cm^2 at the target area. Laser around the joint line and osteotomy site. Repeat twice weekly. PEMFT 20 minutes twice weekly set for pain relief (see manufacturers' instructions).

Manual therapies. Joint compressions five repetitions twice daily. Grade 1 and 2 joint mobilisations three repetitions twice daily (Chapter 5).

Therapeutic exercise. PROM, (Fig. 8.17–8, 8.23–4, 8.15–16) core stability and reversal of muscle loss.

Pain relief. NSAIDS.

Exercise. 10 minutes on lead on level even ground. No games or playing with other dogs, and no stairs.

Modalities. Laser and PEMFT weekly using setting as for days 1–14. Introduce hydrotherapy. Hydrotherapy twice weekly. If using UWTM, start with 4-minute sessions with water above the stifle. Gradually build the session length to 10 minutes. If using pool, perform therapeutic exercises on platforms and start assisted swimming. Gradually build to 10 minutes free swimming.

Manual therapies. Continue joint compressions as above. Move onto Grade 3 joint mobilisations, three repetitions twice daily.

Therapeutic exercise. Biscuits from Hips (Fig. 8.29) 10 repetitions twice daily to both sides. Sit to Stand (Fig. 8.38–9) 10 repetitions twice daily. Rebounding (Fig. 8.76) 2 minutes twice daily. 3 Leg Standing Back Leg (Fig. 8.62) 30 seconds twice daily. Wobble Cushion (Fig. 8.82) for 1 minute twice daily gradually increasing to 5 minutes twice daily.

Days 31–60

Focus for management. Strengthening.

Pain relief. NSAIDS.

Exercise. 20–30 minutes lead exercise twice daily. Introduce mild and moderate gradients. Introduce stairs. No games or playing with other dogs.

Modalities. Laser and PEMFT weekly, settings as mentioned above. Continue with weekly hydrotherapy gradually increasing session length to 20 minutes.

Manual therapies. Joint mobilisations as required.

Therapeutic exercise. As per days 15–30, but increase repetitions by 50%.

Days 61–90

Focus for management. Further strengthening and return to normal activity.

Pain relief. NSAIDS as required.

Exercise. 30–45 minutes lead walk. Off lead for 15 minutes. Introduce steep hills. Traverse as well as going up and down. Gentle ball games. 5 minutes playing with other dogs.

Modalities. As per days 31–60.

Therapeutic exercise. As per days 31–60, but increase repetitions by 50%.

Hock

Achilles tendinopathy

This condition is most commonly seen in Labrador Retrievers. The combined tendon of the gastrocnemius muscles starts to detach from the calcaneus. Aetiology is unknown.

Signalment. Mild to severe lameness with a plantigrade stance. The digits may be clawed. This is due to the fact that the flexor tendons are still intact but now have a greater distance to travel and flex the digits. A thickening may be felt in the tendon.

Diagnosis. Diagnostic ultrasound, X-ray and MRI.

Treatment. These cases are best managed surgically with investigation, debridement and reattachment of the tendon as required. The surgical site is then protected with the hock in extension. This is done using a screw from calcaneus into the tibia, an external fixator or splinting device. Instillation of platelet-rich plasma and/or stem cells directly into the tendon may be of benefit.

Some cases due to other health issues, finance or owner's wishes may be treated conservatively. Again platelet-rich plasma and stems cell may be of use. These dogs are then fitted with a brace, preferably custom made (see Chapter 9). The dog will probably need to wear the brace for the rest of its life.

Surgical post-operative management

Days 1–5

Focus for management. Pain relief. Wound management.

Pain relief. NSAIDS +/− opiates.

Environment. Check flooring and access points. Introduce rugs, runners and ramps as required.

Diet. Weight loss as required.

Exercise. 5 minutes on lead on even level ground. No games or playing with other dogs, and no stairs.

Modalities. Icing 10 minutes twice daily for first 5 days. Shockwave can also be used on day 1, and 600-1500 600 shocks over the length of the tendon and muscle junction.

Laser 8 j/cm^2 at the target area. Repeat twice daily. PEMFT set for increasing vascularisation (see manufacturers' instructions) twice weekly (Chapter 5).

Therapeutic exercise. PROM, flexion and extension of digits (Fig. 8.15-16). Three repetitions twice daily.

Days 6–60

Focus for management. Protection of the operation site.

Pain relief. NSAIDS as required.

Exercise. 10 minutes twice daily on lead. No stairs. No games or playing with other dogs.

Modalities. Repeat shockwave on days 14 and 28. Continue laser and PEMFT weekly.

Therapeutic exercise. As per days 1–5.

Days 61–90

The external fixator and/or screw are normally removed around this time. If using an articulated brace, the degree of movement in the brace can be gradually increased.

Focus for management. Protection of the operation site.

Exercise. This is gradually increased from 10 minutes twice daily to 30 minutes twice daily. Initially, the walking is on flat ground but gentle gradients are then introduced. No stairs. No games or playing with other dogs.

Modalities. Laser and PEMFT weekly.

Therapeutic exercise. Wobble Cushion (Fig. 8.82) initially 1 minute twice daily building to 5 minutes twice daily. Sit to Stand (Fig. 8.38-9) 10 repetitions twice daily.

The non-weight bearing/skipping small terrier-type dog

Signalment. Usually a Parsons Jack Russell Terrier or similar breed that is unwilling to use a back leg after injury and/or surgery. These dogs may be completely non-weight bearing or in mild cases skip occasionally. They will be able to run at speed but only using three legs.

Treatment. First establish if there is a surgical problem. Does the dog have Legg Perthes disease? If the dog has had a femoral head, osteotomy has a bone spur been left that is rubbing on the pelvis? If the dog has had surgery for a luxating patella, are the implants causing a problem? Is the patella still luxating? If the dog has had a cranial cruciate rupture, has it now developed a meniscal injury? If the dog has cruciate surgery, is the implant interfering with the tracking of the patella? Dogs with any of the above are likely to require surgical intervention. The possibility of lumbosacral issues should also be considered. If none of the above is applicable, then the following techniques can be utilised in an attempt to get the dog to use the leg.

Pain relief. NSAIDS as required.

Modalities. Hydrotherapy to strengthen muscles. Start with water at hip height and have the dog walk slowly for 3 minutes. Gradually build up time and reduce depth of water if using UWTM. Start short sessions of swimming and carry out the following therapeutic exercises.

Therapeutic exercise. Passive ROM exercises to all joints in the leg three repetitions twice daily. Parastanding 1 Book (Fig. 8.58) If the dog will not put the foot down to the floor, then bring the floor to the dog by placing books to the required height so as to have the foot touching the top book. Now do Rebounding (Fig. 8.76) exercise to force weight bearing. Repeat for 2 minutes twice daily. Tap the quadriceps and hamstring muscle while the dog is weight bearing. Over time, gradually lower the height of the books to encourage more leg extension. These exercises can be done in water either in the pool with platforms or in the UWTM but using bricks or blocks instead of books.

Try taping a pen cap to the bottom of the weight-bearing back leg. Repeat the rebounding exercise.

Other exercises of benefit. Either on the books or once the dog has started to toe touch. 3 Leg Standing Back Leg (Fig. 8.62). Lift the weight-bearing back leg and hold until the dog becomes uncomfortable. Repeat three times twice daily. This can then progress to lifting the front leg on the same side as the affected leg in addition to the good back leg Parastanding (Fig. 8.63).

Motor sequencing. Sometimes these dogs have inappropriate motor sequencing. Before weight is switched onto the affected leg, the leg muscles and core muscles must fire in preparation for loading. To encourage motor sequencing, alternately lift and push down on the dogs legs in a marching fashion. Tap or tickle the abdominal muscles on the affected side just as the leg is about to bear weight. This will take two people. Continue for 2 minutes twice daily. Again the exercise can also be performed in water.

Osteoarthritis

Osteoarthritis in the dog is a progressive disease. The disease changes as it progresses and calls for a multimodal approach to management. Much of the OA seen is dogs is due to conformation defects such as cruciate disease, elbow and hip dysplasia. Dogs with OA limp for one of three reasons that may occur singularly or in combination: pain, reduced range of motion and muscle weakness. For instance, range of motion is very important in dogs with elbow OA. If there is reduced ROM, the dog cannot extend the leg sufficiently and will limp. The joint may also be painful, contributing further to the lameness. In the hip, ROM is less important as the dog can propel the back leg forward using the paraspinal muscles and increased stifle and hock flexion and extension. However, muscle mass is important in the hip joint and any wasting will make movement difficult even if the pain is controlled. The focus for management of OA is pain relief and mobility. Bearing this in mind then allows us to focus our management strategies. Professor Stuart Carmichael of Surrey University and director of Fitzpatrick Referrals, Surrey, devised the AIMOA system for arthritis management (www.aimoasys.com). This is the system that we use, with great success, in our clinic (Figure 11.12).

The AIMOA system is based on five areas for management.

A for Analgesia.

B for Body condition score and diet.

C for Care from both an environmental perspective and a toxicity perspective with the long-term use of pain relief medication.

D for Disease modification.

E for Exercise.

Also added to these areas is F for Follow-up. A lot of OA cases are seen only for medication checks and often have deteriorated significantly between visits. Monitoring and adjustment of the management plan is key to extending and improving the lives of these animals. Remember a dog off its legs is one of the most common reasons for euthanasia.

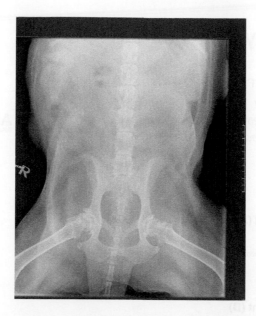

Figure 11.12   Radiograph of a dog with advanced osteoarthritis of the hips. In osteoarthritis, there is poor correlation between radiological finding and degree of lameness. This particular dog leads a very active life and was able to go for two 45-minute walks every day.

A – Analgesia. NSAIDS form the core of any pain relief program. They are effective and available in different forms. In OA, there is background pain punctuated by spikes of more severe pain. As veterinarians, we have been guilty in the past of only treating the spikes and ignoring the background pain. We run OA clinics at our centre and if we get the analgesia correct, the first thing an owner reports is a change in dog's demeanour. They report that their dog is happier and more active. We will then see an improvement in the limping and stiffness.

Often NSAIDS therapy is stopped very early in the belief that it is going to cause gut bleeding or renal problems. Whilst these side effects do occur, they are not as frequent as may be believed. For dogs that are NSAID-intolerant, the adjuncts below should be used. Another alternative is acupuncture.

If NSAIDS alone are not managing the pain, then adjuncts such as acetaminophen (paracetamol) or tramadol can be added. If there are signs of local or central sensitisation, then further adjuncts such as gabapentin or amantadine can also be added.

Omega 3 fish oils and eicosapentaenoic acid (EPA) in particular also help with long-term pain control in chronic OA patients.

For more details on pain and pain regulation, see Chapter 10.

B – Body condition score. Obesity and excess weight are significant contributing factors in OA. The key to the success of any weight-loss plan is to keep the owner motivated. Ideally a dog should lose 0.5–1% body weight per week. However, it takes 6–9% body weight loss before any improvement is seen in osteoarthritic dogs. This means that the owners have to stay motivated for at least 6 weeks before there is any improvement in clinical signs.

AIM-OA Sys
Veterinary Monitoring

ARTHRITIS CARE PLAN (AIM-OA)

Prepared for: Harvey

Prepared on: 25/09/2014 13:22:48

(Printed: 25/09/2014 13:27:28)

Weight: 30.70 Kg

A ◯◯●
B ◯◯◯
C ◯◯● AIM-OA Sys
Veterinary Monitoring
D ◯◯◯
E ●◯◯

CARE INSTRUCTIONS

Pain Management (A)

◯◯●

NSAID 1 plus Omega 3 Previcox (Firocoxib)

NOTES:

Joint Improvement (D)

◯◯◯

Reference:H laser hydrotherapy joint mobilisations

NOTES:

Dietary Advice (B)

◯◯◯

Recommended Food: Hills J/D Light EPA 40mg/kg/day 1200mg/day

NOTES:

Exercise Guidelines (E)

●◯◯

Reference:8 Off lead in house when owner present.20 minutes walk twice daily. 5 minutes off lead Hill work No games, or playing with others dogs Recommended Exercises: 19,20,23,24,25,26,27,31,32,34,35, 36,37,38,39,40,41,42,43,45

NOTES:

Help sheets and comments (C)

◯◯●

Care Flags: 1:Advise rugs and runners 2:Care with medication 1:It is advisable to install rugs and runners to reduce impact joints from laminate or slippery flooring. 2:Caution with medication. May need regular blood/urine samples. Consider medication.

NOTES:

Follow up

Figure 11.13   Printout for owner of the AIMOA system for arthritis management in dogs. The traffic lights highlight the focus for management.

C – Care. When prescribing NSAIDS, it is important to make owners aware of any potential side effects. Gastric and intestinal irritation and ulceration are the most commonly reported problems causing vomiting and diarrhoea. Some dogs may have occult bleeding from the gut or may pass black motions. Other potential side effects are to the kidneys and liver. Any dog put on long-term NSAIDS should have routine blood work.

Care is also for care in the environment. Simple aids such as ramps and harnesses (see Chapter 9) can make the management of these cases much easier for both dog and owner. Similarly, rugs and runners reduce the risk of falls and exacerbations on slippery flooring.

D – Disease. In this section are things that can influence the progression of the disease. These would include things such as the addition of EPA to the diet. Other things to consider would be platelet-rich plasma and stem cells. Again the timing of these interventions would need careful planning. Surgery would also come into this box. For instance, for the treatment of carpal OA, a pancarpal arthrodesis is one option with good results. Similarly, in the management of hip, dysplasia can be treated with joint replacement.

Other things that should also be considered are physiotherapy techniques such as joint mobilisations and joint compressions (Chapter 6). These will help maintain or even improve ROM and joint health. Modalities such as laser will help with pain relief while hydrotherapy will also aid analgesia. It will also help maintain or improve muscle mass (Chapter 5).

E – Exercise. It is important to keep the OA dogs mobile as much as possible. If these dogs are just rested, then range of motion and muscle mass will be lost. A suitable exercise regime should be worked out for each dog remembering that this will change as the dog progresses through the disease. Also, a home exercise program will help maintain ROM and muscle mass.

An example of the AIMOA printout sheet is shown. The scores for each box are derived from an owner and veterinarian survey, the answers of which are then processed through a complex algorithm. This produces advice for each area of management. The system then uses a traffic light system to demonstrate which are the main areas for focus (Figure 11.13). The surveys are repeated at regular intervals and a different range of suggestions is made depending on how the dog is responding to treatment.

CHAPTER 12

Setting up a physiotherapy clinic

When setting up a physiotherapy clinic, the first consideration is whether it is to be in-house and incorporated within the existing practice buildings or a stand-alone venue.

There are advantages and disadvantages for both alternatives.

In-house versus stand-alone

In-house

Pros
Reduced overheads

By using the same buildings, there is an obvious financial benefit as the facility can use the same reception and waiting areas.

Existing consult rooms can be used for clinical examination and some treatments, such as manual therapies, laser and ultrasound. Remember that most examinations and treatments are carried out on mats on the floor, and hence there must be sufficient space in the existing consult room for these (Figure 12.1(a) and (b)). Other treatments such as poles and cones and physio balls are going to need extra space that has to be accommodated within the existing buildings. Furthermore, the addition of a pool or underwater treadmill will require further (ground floor) space. Consideration will also have to be given to strength of flooring and access to install the hydrotherapy unit.

Another pro of in-house is that it can *utilise existing staff*. This is particularly so of reception staff that can make appointments, answer the telephone and take payments. It may also be possible to adjust veterinarian and nurse rotas so as to make efficient use of professional time.

Neurological cases, such as IVDD, may be able to make use of *existing kennels*, so that multiple short treatment sessions can be carried out throughout the day (Figure 12.2(a) and (b)). These dogs tire very quickly, and fatigue is a major consideration during the rehabilitation of these dogs. Also bladder and bowel management is better carried out under veterinary supervision and where catheters and so on are available.

Equipment such as the laser can be used on other cases, for example, otitis externa and granulating wounds. In the stand-alone situation, the laser would be at a different location.

Practical Physiotherapy for Small Animal Practice, First Edition.
Edited by David Prydie and Isobel Hewitt.
© 2015 John Wiley & Sons, Ltd. Published 2015 by John Wiley & Sons, Ltd.
Companion Website: www.wiley.com/go/practical-physiotherapy-for-small-animals

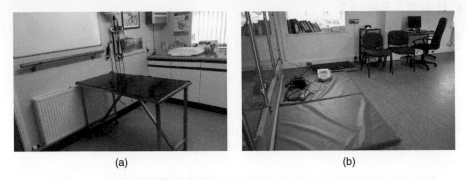

(a)   (b)

Figure 12.1   (a) and (b) Traditional consult rooms may not have enough room to accommodate mats on the floor for examination and treatment.

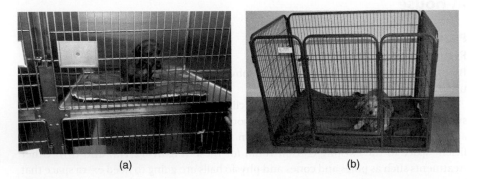

(a)   (b)

Figure 12.2   (a) and (b) Existing kennels can be used for in patients that need bladder management. However, collapsible kennels can fulfil the same task and maintain flexibility of floor space.

Cons

In-house referrals only. It is unlikely that neighbouring practices will refer to the premises of a competitor. Business expansion will be restricted to in-house referrals only.

Extra pressure will be put on current buildings and staff. Is there a quiet period when physiotherapy appointments could be fitted in? Will clients want to come in at the quiet period? There is a reason why it is a quiet period.

Patients may be stressed in the waiting area. Remember this is the place the dog comes to get its vaccinations and anal glands emptied.

Stand-alone

Pros

Away from the hustle of the main practice. The atmosphere is less clinical, and clients and patients are more likely to be able to relax, which makes treatment much easier.

May attract outside referrals. Because the premises are not directly linked to an existing practice, there is the possibility of attracting referrals from neighbouring practices.

A building can be selected that is suitable for purpose or adapted for purpose. The space may allow for a hydrotherapy suite as well as treatment rooms and exercise areas.

Cons
Additional overheads. A stand-alone building will obviously attract its own rent and rates as well as heating and lighting costs.

Staffing. More staff will be required to man reception, answer the phone and so on, as well as the treatment personnel.

Extra space may be required for day *kennelling* of spinal patients. For a lot of the time, this space may be unused.

Space requirements

These apply to areas that are required/desired in both an in-house and stand-alone operation. Obviously, in the stand–alone, some of these rooms may already exist.

Individual rooms
Waiting room
A minimum space of 70 sq. ft. (6.5 m²) will be required. With a good appointment system and therapists that run to time, the waiting room should only have to accommodate one patient with two or three owners at any one time. If possible, it should be able to have a small retail stand stocked with diets relevant to rehab, for example, weight loss diets, mobility diets, supplements, harnesses and other physiotherapy aids. Obviously, in the in-house situation, the waiting room will already be in existence and likely to be considerably larger.

Treatment room
In the in-house situation, this will double as a consult room and the size will be predetermined. Whilst treatments such as laser and ultrasound can be performed in a small room of 70 sq. ft. or less, cone and pole work will need a much larger space (Figure 12.3). In the new or stand-alone unit, the size would be a minimum of 200 sq. ft. (18.5 m²), preferably larger. It may be possible to utilise a corridor or passageway for some of these activities, provided they do not stop the traffic flow of the practice.

UWTM
The minimum space requirement for an underwater treadmill is about 200 sq. ft. minimum. There must be room for the dogs to access the treadmill at either end with the doors fully open. An area is required for drying the dogs and ideally an area to shower them before and after their treatment. There will also need to be space for the filters and pumps as well as the holding tank(s) (Figure 12.4).

The floor will need to be substantial enough to support the weight of the UWTM when filled with water. Easy access to the space where the treadmill is to be situated

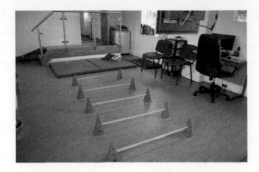

Figure 12.3 A treatment room with cones and poles will require more space than a traditional consult room.

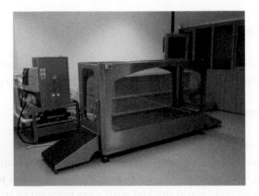

Figure 12.4 Underwater treadmill suite with room for shower, holding tank and pump housing.

is essential. These are very heavy pieces of equipment that have to be wheeled into position. The treadmill unit itself is over 6.5 ft (2 m) in length [9.5 ft (3 m) with the doors open]. The width is approximately 2.3 ft (0.7 m). The width of access doors will need to be checked carefully. Turning corners requires a lot more space than may have been anticipated.

Pool

I would suggest that even a small pool would require a minimum area of 400 sq. ft. (37.1 m²). There must be sufficient space for pumps and filters as well as a shower area. If the pool is above ground, then there needs to be enough space for entry and exit ramps. Again the suitability and strength of the floor should be checked (Figure 12.5).

Some above-ground pools come as a preformed fibre glass/resin moulding. In this case, access will be critical. Most above-ground pools are now assembled on site, hence access is less of an issue.

Below-ground pools are likely to require vehicular access as well as substantially more space than above-ground pools. A separate plant room with heat exchanger and humidifier is often required for larger pools (Figure 12.6).

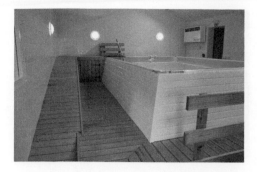

Figure 12.5   Space for even a modest pool will need careful consideration to accommodate entry and exit ramps.

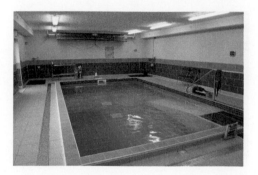

Figure 12.6   Below-ground pools will need consideration for plant machinery and vehicle access.

Equipment

A physiotherapy clinic can be established with very little investment. High-ticket price items, such as the laser, UWTM or pool, are not essential for getting started.

I have tried to give some indication of cost of each of the items using the $ sign.

$ = small kitchen electrical item, $$ = meal for two people at a good restaurant, $$$ = a weekend break for two people, $$$$ = price of a luxury holiday for two people, $$$$$ = the price of a family saloon car or more.

Must have pieces of equipment
Goniometers $
Set of three different sizes to accommodate different breeds and different joints. There are different styles and it is really down to operator preference.

Tip: Try to get goniometers with a white background for the numbers. These are far easier to read, especially against the background of a dark dog (Figure 12.7).

Girthometer or Gulick $
These are a type of tape measure for measuring muscle girth.

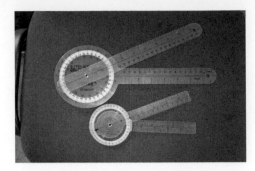

Figure 12.7 Goniometers with white backgrounds make readings easier.

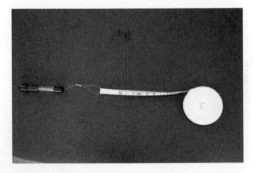

Figure 12.8 Gulicks or girthometers have a spring-loaded tensioning device that gives more repeatable results.

Tip: Try to find a girthometer that has the spring-loaded device. These are a little more expensive than a tape measure but are far more consistent with readings (Figure 12.8).

Mats $$

A lot of procedures will be carried out on the floor. Deep-fill waterproof mats are ideal for working on (Figure 12.9).

Gel packs/freezer packs $

These need to be flexible to wrap around joints. Gel packs or freezer packs with lots of small pockets are easiest for this. The cold pack should not come into direct contact with the animal (Figure 12.10).

The gel packs can be used to deliver heat therapy as well as cooling. Alternatively, a damp flannel heated in the microwave will suffice.

Tip: Remember wet heat is more effective than dry heat. Therefore, a hot wet flannel reheated several times will be more effective than a wheat bag or heat mat.

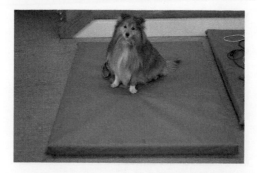

Figure 12.9   Deep-fill wipe clean mats are ideal for examination and treatment.

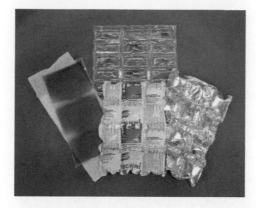

Figure 12.10   Keep a selection of gel packs in the freezer. Make sure you have sufficient time to replenish cold applications rather than having to wait for the gel packs to cool again.

Wobble cushion $

These are items that the owner should be encouraged to purchase for home use with his/her animal. They are inexpensive and widely available on the Internet (Figure 12.11).

Tip: Try not to loan out equipment, because it has a habit of not being returned.

Wobble board $

These are available commercially or can be easily fabricated. Try to have unidirectional and multidirectional boards (Figure 12.12).

Plastic models of joints $$

These are essential for explaining clinical findings to clients (Figure 12.13).

Tip: Many of the pharmaceutical companies give these away as promotional items. You will still have to buy the joints missing from your collection.

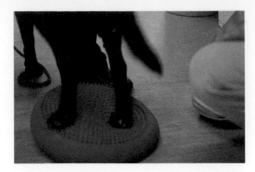

Figure 12.11   Wobble cushions are readily available on the Internet.

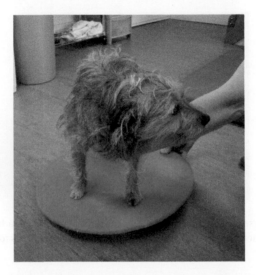

Figure 12.12   Wobble boards. These are available from physio suppliers or can be easily fabricated.

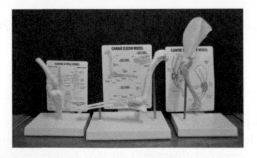

Figure 12.13   Plastic models of joints are essential for explaining to clients what is wrong with their pet.

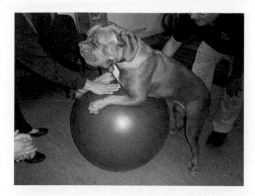

Figure 12.14   A range of physio balls and peanuts is required to accommodate the different sizes of patients.

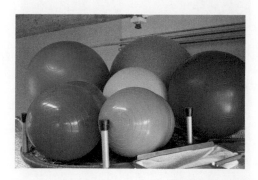

Figure 12.15   Storage of physio balls and peanuts can be challenging. On top of a UWTM holding tank or above kennels do not use up valuable floor space.

Physio balls and peanuts $–$$

You will need a selection of sizes of these for different breeds. Storage can be a problem as they are very bulky (Figure 12.14). On top of a UWTM storage tank is a good place. Try to keep the balls and peanuts fully inflated (Figure 12.15). It is possible to let air out of the ball during a session if the height is wrong for a particular patient.

Tip: Make sure you buy the tough anti-burst balls rather than the cheaper Pilates balls. The dog's nails and dewclaws will burst these.

Theraband™ tubing $

The tubing is easier to use than the Pilates bands. The tubing comes in a variety of strengths depicted by a different colour. For dog use, the ultra-thin (beige), thin (yellow) and medium (red) will suffice (Figure 12.16).

Hair scrunchies $

These are widely available from supermarkets or pharmacies. Keep a range of sizes in stock to accommodate different-sized dogs (Figure 12.17).

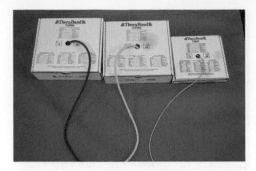

Figure 12.16 Theraband™ tubes are useful way of adding resistance to exercises as well as providing inward or outward rotation of the back legs.

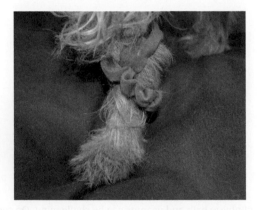

Figure 12.17 Hair scrunchies are an easy cost-effective way to stimulate sensation.

Cones and poles $–$$

Various cone and pole sets are available on the Internet. Specific dog sets are also available (Figure 12.18).

Tip: Plumbing waste pipe can be used for the poles. A coloured tape spiralled around the pole will enhance visibility. The loop part of hook and loop (Velcro) can be wrapped around the ends of each pole. The hook part of the hook and look can then be applied down the height of traffic cones. The poles can then be stuck onto the cones at an appropriate height for each patient (Figure 12.19).

Electric muscle stimulation $

This is another unit that I encourage owners to purchase rather than loan. The units are freely available on the Internet and are not expensive. The sticky pads are consumable items (Figure 12.20).

Tip: Keep spare pads in stock. Alternatively reusable rubber pads are available. They are a bit more expensive than the adhesive pads but can be cleaned and reused. Tape may be needed to hold them in place. Use ultrasound gel to ensure a good skin contact (Figure 12.21).

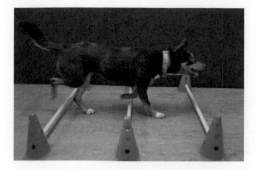

Figure 12.18   Various sets of cones and poles are available, some specifically made for canine rehabilitation.

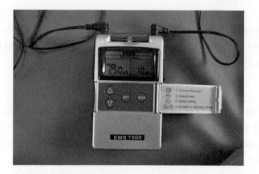

Figure 12.19   Velcro applied to traffic cones and poles provides a solid, easily adjusted system.

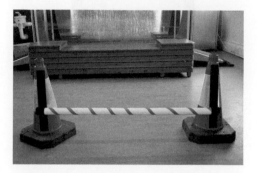

Figure 12.20   EMS machines are readily available on the Internet. Encourage owners to buy their own.

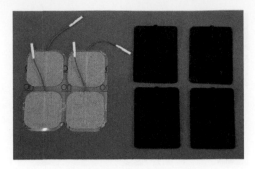

Figure 12.21 EMS pads come as disposable sticky pads or more expensive reusable rubber pads.

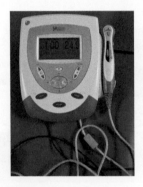

Figure 12.22 Typical Class 3b laser.

Next pieces of equipment to buy
Lasers
These are an important piece of equipment, but not essential. They have the advantage over ultrasound in that the patient does not have to be shaved or covered in gel. They are, however, more expensive than ultrasound machines.

Class 3b $$$$
A variety of Class 3b lasers are available. They all come with interchangeable heads that feature one or more laser diodes and LED clusters. Protective glasses are usually included. The amount of laser energy will need to be calculated for each patient and will be based on coat colour, weight and depth of target tissue. Once these have been calculated the first few times, the operator usually learns the required settings (Figure 12.22).

Class 4 $$$$$
These machines are quite an investment and need carefully worked out financial strategy. The area where the machine is to be used will need to be carefully selected due to health and safety regulations applied to these machines. Settings can be preselected based again on coat colour, weight and target area (Figure 12.23).

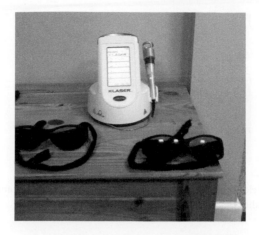

Figure 12.23   Typical Class 4 laser.

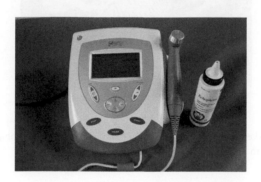

Figure 12.24   Ultrasound machine. Make sure to purchase a machine with 1 and 3.3MHz settings.

Ultrasound $$$

These machines are a useful addition to the armoury. They are particularly useful for deep heating (continuous mode) or for tendon issues (pulsed mode) (Figure 12.24).

Tip: Make sure you buy a machine that has 1 and 3.3 MHz settings. Some machines only come with 1 MHz setting. The extra setting is usually available for the same price or only a little more.

Pulsed electromagnetic field therapy $$

This is a useful piece of equipment that can be used whilst administering other treatments. The patient just has to sit on the mat or within the magnetic field (Figure 12.25).

Tip: Make sure you have a static magnet at hand to demonstrate the pulsing effect to clients.

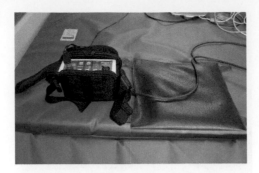

Figure 12.25 Pulsed electromagnetic field therapy units are inexpensive and treatment can be administered while other treatments are being conducted.

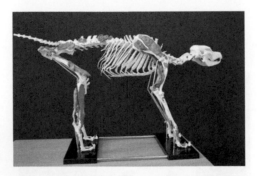

Figure 12.26 A full skeleton is the next thing on from joint models and helps demonstrate the location of problems to owners.

Skeleton $$

Useful for demonstrating areas of treatment on the whole dog rather than restricted to one area (Figure 12.26).

Trampette $–$$

Specialist physiotherapy trampettes can be quite expensive. Children's trampettes can be used although the springs are much stiffer (Figure 12.27).

Air mattress $

These are another inexpensive tool for core stability and proprioception work (Figure 12.28).

Tip: Be sure to buy the thicker fabric covered mattresses as bursting with sharp nails is a real problem.

Land treadmill $$–$$$

There are several companies making specialist dog treadmills. With sides and cut–outs, it is possible to use a human treadmill but the dogs will have to be trained to use this and not jump off the side (Figure 12.29).

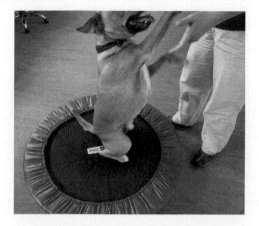

Figure 12.27 Specialist physiotherapy trampettes are costly. Children's trampettes work OK but the springs have more tension and need a bit of use to soften up.

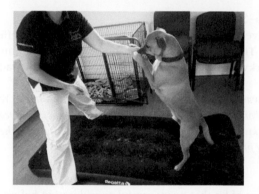

Figure 12.28 Be sure to purchase the tougher flock covered air mattress to avoid bursting by claws.

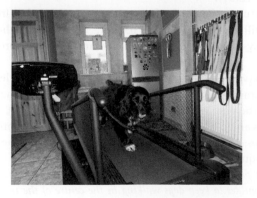

Figure 12.29 Land treadmills should have sides and ideally an automatic cut-off system.

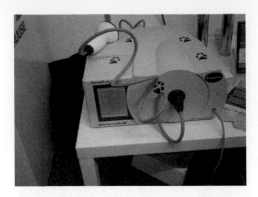

Figure 12.30 Shockwave is very useful piece of kit and could be hired from a neighbouring equine practice.

Tip: Make sure the treadmill inclines and can run in forward and backward directions.

Shockwave $$$$–$$$$$

Some less-expensive models of shockwave that use the Piezo effect have recently become available. These new machines do not require the animal to be sedated. However, the shockwave that they deliver is much less than traditional machines (Figure 12.30).

Tip: Some shockwave manufacturers/distributors run a hire scheme. You arrange for your patients to come in all on a particular day. The shockwave machine is shipped to you the previous day. You use the shockwave on your patients. You ship the machine back the following day. You are charged shipping plus the number of shocks that you have used.

UWTM $$$$$

This is another piece of kit that needs careful consideration before buying. Not only does space and flooring have to be taken into account but also staffing. To justify purchase, the treadmill needs to be in daily use. There is also the staffing issue to be considered (Figure 12.31).

Some manufactures offer a 'freshwater' system. With this freshwater, heated water is used to fill the tank for each patient. The water is then flushed down the drain. These systems are environmentally unsound and probably financially unsound.

Most systems have a holding tank or tanks. The water is recycled. It is cleaned by passing through some sort of filter, heated and held in the holding tank(s). If a pool is also fitted, then the pool water can act as the reservoir for the UWTM.

With both pools and UWTMs, good water management is essential to prevent contamination and cross infection. Intraday, daily and weekly regimes will be required to maintain water quality.

Tip: Float tubes or 'noodles' available from most pool supply shops and beach front vendors make good guides to keep dogs walking in the centre of the treadmill conveyor belt (Figure 12.32).

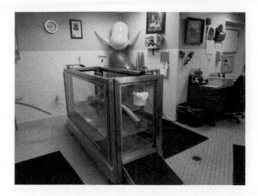

Figure 12.31   The UWTM is a substantial financial commitment and the business case needs to be carefully considered.

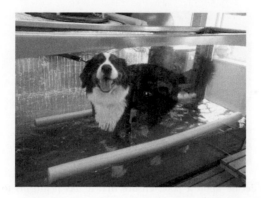

Figure 12.32   Float noodles are a good way to keep dogs in the centre of the UWTM.

Tip: Make sure with the machine you purchase it is possible to lift the belt assembly to clean underneath. In the warm water, grime builds up rapidly here and at least daily cleaning is required (Figure 12.33).

Pool $$$$–$$$$$

Again as with the underwater treadmill, this is a purchase that must be properly budgeted for. Particular attention needs to be paid to the running costs for the heating (or cooling) of the water. These can be quite substantial in cooler climates. Another consideration is staffing. Usually, staff will have to change into wetsuits to accompany the dog in the pool. Changing rooms and staff showers will be required. Time will also have to be allocated for changing. Once in a wetsuit, it may be difficult for a staff member to carry out other duties such as lasering.

Be aware that a lot of start-up rehab units that have fitted both a pool and a UWTM have ended up taking the pool out because of running cost. They also found they used the UWTM a lot more than the pool given the choice.

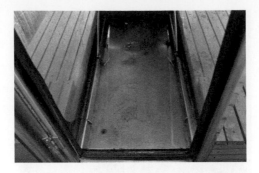

Figure 12.33 Grit from dogs' feet and grime rapidly build up in the warm watery environment of the UWTM. Try to ensure that the machine you chose can be thoroughly cleaned, even under the belt.

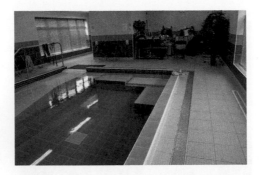

Figure 12.34 If you decide upon a pool, ensure that it has platforms to allow therapeutic exercises to be done in the water.

Tip: Try to incorporate submerged platforms of various heights in the pool design (Figure 12.34). This will allow manual therapies to be carried out in the water as well as simply swimming the patients. Also try to build in resistance jets.

Float coats and buoyancy aids $–$$

If you decide to offer hydrotherapy, then float coats and buoyancy aids are essential. A range of sizes from XXS to XXL will be required (Figure 12.35).

Staffing and charging

Initial assessment should be carried out by either a veterinarian trained in physiotherapy or a physiotherapist trained in canine orthopaedic conditions. The initial examination will take at least 1 hour and sometimes substantially longer. The examining clinician works out a treatment plan. This plan is implemented at follow-up visits. A veterinary nurse or physio-assistant who has had suitable training conducts these sessions. Typically these last 30–45 minutes. Reassessment sessions by the veterinarian or

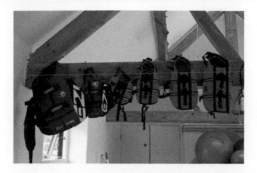

Figure 12.35   A range of types and sizes of buoyancy aids will be required for any hydrotherapy unit.

physiotherapist should happen at regular intervals, such as 3 weeks, where a revised plan can be drawn up. The revised plan is then once again implemented by the nurse or physio-assistant.

Charges can be based on a higher fee for a veterinarian/physiotherapist initial assessments and follow-up sessions. A separate (lower) fee is applied for nurse/physio-assistant sessions. These sessions can be based on an hourly rate or a fixed fee per session.

Laser, ultrasound, pulsed and PEMFT are charged for minutes in addition to session charges. Shockwave is charged per shock plus the session time plus the sedation, if required.

The annual sales figure for a physiotherapy unit will be much lower than in traditional veterinary practice. However, there is little or no drugs bill, hence the gross margin will be much higher. As with veterinary practice, keeping control of staffing costs is the key to financial success.

APPENDIX 1

Nomenclature

This may seem basic but it is important to accurately describe the location of any problem areas. Terms such as anterior, posterior, superior and inferior should be avoided, as these are terms applicable to the upright human body.

Cranial	towards the head of the animal
Caudal	towards the tail of the animal
Dorsal	towards the top surface of the animal
Ventral	towards the bottom surface of the animal
Lateral	towards the outside of the animal
Medial	towards the centre of the animal
Proximal	nearer the body
Distal	further away from the body
Abduction	to take away from the body
Adduction	to bring towards the body
Rostral	towards the nose (used for describing structures on the head)
Palmer surface	the ventral surface of the front feet
Planter surface	the ventral surface of the back feet
Rotation	to twist around a central axis
Circumduction	circular or conical movement of a body part or limb. It involves flexion, extension, adduction and abduction.
Supination	to turn the palmer or planter surface inwards and upwards
Pronation	to turn the palmer or planter surface outwards and downwards
Flexion	to bend a joint bringing the limb closer to the body
Extension	to straighten a joint taking the limb away from the body
Atrophy	reduction in size
Hypertrophy	increase in size
Acute	sudden or recent in onset
Chronic	long-standing
itis	meaning inflammation of, for example, septic arthritis
Opathy	little or no inflammation but still a problem, for example, tendinopathy

Practical Physiotherapy for Small Animal Practice, First Edition.
Edited by David Prydie and Isobel Hewitt.
© 2015 John Wiley & Sons, Ltd. Published 2015 by John Wiley & Sons, Ltd.
Companion Website: www.wiley.com/go/practical-physiotherapy-for-small-animals

APPENDIX 2

Regenerative medicine

In the last few years, the use of platelet-rich plasma and stem cells has become more commonplace in small animal practice.

Platelet-rich plasma (PRP)

Platelets have long been associated with blood clotting. However, platelets also contain a vast array of growth factors involved in healing. These include platelet-derived growth factors (PDGF), β-thromboglobulin, fibroblast growth factor, insulin-like growth factor 1, epidermal growth factor and vascular endothelial growth factor. These growth factors recruit and differentiate progenitor cells promoting angiogenesis and vascularisation, tissue repair and replenishment of the extracellular matrix.

The technique for use involves the collection of blood from the dog, in vitro concentration of the platelets and re-injection of the PRP into the target tissue or joint. There are several techniques for concentrating the platelets and marketed by different companies. Some use a filtration method to remove the red blood cells from the whole blood (e.g. PET, PALL Corporation). Others separate the red blood cells from the platelets by centrifuging the whole blood (e.g. Arthrex ACP® Double Syringe System).

The volume of blood taken from the patient depends upon the size of the patient, the target tissue or joint and whether the procedure will be repeated.

PRP therapy appears to be of most benefit if used early in the course of a disease. It has been used with successful results in osteoarthritis, tendinopathies and medial shoulder instabilities.

Stem cells therapy (SCT)

There are currently two methods available for harvesting stem cells in the dog. The first method involves the harvesting of fat, usually from the falciform ligament, which is sent to the processing laboratory where it is chopped, rinsed and broken down by collagenase enzymes. The resultant soup is centrifuged and the cellular residue is resuspended and sent back to the veterinary surgeon for injection into the target tissue or joint. This method probably produces adipose-derived stromal cells with multipotent differentiation capabilities. There is no expansion of a cellular linage and

Practical Physiotherapy for Small Animal Practice, First Edition.
Edited by David Prydie and Isobel Hewitt.
© 2015 John Wiley & Sons, Ltd. Published 2015 by John Wiley & Sons, Ltd.
Companion Website: www.wiley.com/go/practical-physiotherapy-for-small-animals

this product is more accurately referred to as stromal vascular fraction (SVF) rather than stem cells.

The second method of producing stem cells is by collecting bone marrow or adipose tissue which undergoes a process similar to the above. The sample is then cultured to achieve cellular expansion and greater homogenicity. These more uniform and culture expanded cells are then concentrated and resuspended for use. Cells derived from this method are referred to as mesenchymal stromal (MCS) cells rather than stem cells.

Stem cells are being used increasingly in OA and other cases such as those mentioned with PRP. The results are encouraging, but larger, long-term studies are required.

APPENDIX 3
Further reading

Animal Physiotherapy: Assessment, Treatment and Rehabilitation of Animals. Edited by Lesley Goff, Catherine McGowan, Narelle Stubbs. Wiley-Blackwell, 2007.

Canine Rehabilitation & Physical Therapy, 2nd Edition. Darryl L. Millis, David Levine. Saunders, 2013.

Essential Facts of Physiotherapy in Dogs and Cats. Barbara Bockstahler, David Levine, Darryl Millis. BE VetVerlag, 2004.

Canine Sports Medicine and Rehabilitation. Edited by M. Christine Zink, Janet B. Van Dyke. Wiley-Blackwell, 2013.

Successful Practitioners in Canine Rehabilitation and Physiotherapy, Laurie Edge-Hughes. Four Leg Rehab Inc., 2014.

Anatomy and Physiology of Domestic Animals, 2nd Edition. R. Michael Akers, D. Michael Denbow. Wiley-Blackwell, 2013.

Anatomy and Physiology for Veterinary Technicians and Nurses: A Clinical Approach. Robin Sturtz, Lori Asprea. Wiley-Blackwell, 2012.

Miller's Anatomy of the Dog, 4th Edition. Howard E. Evans, Alexander DeLahunta. Elsevier Saunders, 2013.

Textbook of Veterinary Anatomy, 4th Edition. K. M. Dyce, Wolfgang O. Sack, C.J.G. Wensing. Elsevier Health Sciences, 2009.

Color Atlas of Clinical Anatomy of the Dog and Cat, 2nd Edition. J.S. Boyd, C. Paterson, Allan H. May. Mosby, 2001.

Veterinary Neuroanatomy: A Clinical Approach. Christine E. Thomson, Caroline Hahn. Elsevier, 2012.

Pain Management in Veterinary Practice, Edited by Christine M. Egger, Lydia Love, Tom Doherty. Wiley-Blackwell, 2013.

BSAVA Manual of Canine and Feline Anaesthesia and Analgesia, 2nd Edition. Edited by Chris Seymour, Tanya Duke-Novakovski. BSAVA, 2007.

BSAVA Manual of Small Animal Fracture Repair and Management. Edited by Andrew R. Coughlan, Andrew Miller. BSAVA, 1998.

BSAVA Manual of Canine and Feline Rehabilitation, Supportive and Palliative Care. Edited by Samantha Lindley, Penny Watson. BSAVA, 2010.

BSAVA Manual of Canine and Feline Neurology, 3rd Edition. Edited by Simon R. Platt, Natasha J. Olby.BSAVA, 2011.

Practical Physiotherapy for Small Animal Practice, First Edition.
Edited by David Prydie and Isobel Hewitt.
© 2015 John Wiley & Sons, Ltd. Published 2015 by John Wiley & Sons, Ltd.
Companion Website: www.wiley.com/go/practical-physiotherapy-for-small-animals

BSAVA Manual of Canine and Feline Musculoskeletal Disorders. Edited by John E.F. Houlton, James L. Cook, John F. Innes, Sorrel J. Langley-Hobbs. BSAVA, 2006.

Small Animal Bandaging, Casting, and Splinting Techniques. Steven F. Swaim, Walter C. Renberg, Kathy M. Shike. Wiley-Blackwell, 2011.

BSAVA Small Animal Formulary, 8th Edition. Ian Ramsey. BSAVA, 2014.

Veterinary Acupuncture, Ancient Art to Modern Science, 2nd Edition. Allen M. Schoen. Mosby, 2000.

Essentials of Western Veterinary Acupuncture. Samantha Lindley, Mike Cummings. Wiley-Blackwell, 2006.

APPENDIX 4

Useful websites for aids and equipment

Aids, splints and braces

www.dogleggs.com – Shoulder Stabilisation System.

www.handicappedpets.com – products for pets with special needs.

www.helpemup.com – Help 'Em Up Harness.

www.jorvet.com – Jorvet Pet Brace and MB Spinal Brace.

www.orthodog.com – Hip Hound.

www.therapaw.com – Thera-Paw Boots, Tarso-Flex, Dorsi-Flex Assist and Carpo-Flex-X.

www.udsmr.org – Uniform Data System for Medical Rehabilitation.

www.vetinst.com – Biko Physio Brace.

www.canineicer.com – icing/warming wraps.

www.orthovet.com – canine & feline splints & braces.

www.aceorthosolutions.com – stifle, carpal and hock braces.

www.animalorthocare.com – orthotics, prosthetics and other assistive devices.

www.k-9orthotics.com – orthotics, prosthetics and other assistive devices.

www.orthopets.com – custom-made orthotics and braces.

Carts

www.eddieswheels.com

www.k9carts.com

www.dogswheels.com

www.walkinwheels.com

General physiotherapy equipment

www.emeservices.com Physiotherapy supplies and servicing.

www.pattersonmedical.com Physiotherapy equipment and supplies.

Lasers

www.spectravet.com.
www.thorlaser.com.
www.chattanooga.com.
www.klaser.co.uk.
www.k-laserusa.com.
www.respondsystems.com.
www.litecure.com.

Underwater treadmills

www.physio-vet.com.
www.tudortreadmills.com.
www.hudsonaquatic.com.
www.hydrophysio.com.
www.burtonsveterinary.com.
www.animalrehab.co.uk.

Organisations

www.bsava.com British Small Animal Veterinary Association.
www.vsmr.org American College of Veterinary Sports Medicine and Rehabilitation.
www.acpat.org Association of Chartered Physiotherapists in Animal Therapy.
www.ivapm.org International Veterinary Academy of Pain Management.
www.electrotherapy.org Large database of electrotherapy research.

Miscellaneous

www.physio-vet.co.uk Authors website.
www.aimoasys.com Osteoarthritis management website.

Pain scoring charts

www.newmetrica.com/cpms/
http://www.csuanimalcancercenter.org/assets/files/csu_acute_pain_scale_canine.pdf
http://www.biomedcentral.com/content/supplementary/s12917-015-0338-4-s2.pdf

Index

Note: Page numbers in italics represent figures, those in bold represent tables.

Practical Physiotherapy for Small Animal Practice, First Edition.
Edited by David Prydie and Isobel Hewitt.
© 2015 John Wiley & Sons, Ltd. Published 2015 by John Wiley & Sons, Ltd.
Companion Website: www.wiley.com/go/practical-physiotherapy-for-small-animals